GRILLING COOKBOOK

GRILL & GRILL SOMEMORE!

50 Recipes for Grilling Everything You Love

Kara Chambers

Copyright © 2020 Kara Chambers

All Rights Reserved

Copyright 2020 By Kara Chambers - All rights reserved.

The following book is produced below with the goal of providing information that is as accurate and reliable as possible. Regardless, purchasing this eBook can be seen as consent to the fact that both the publisher and the author of this book are in no way experts on the topics discussed within and that any recommendations or suggestions that are made herein are for entertainment purposes only. Professionals should be consulted as needed prior to undertaking any of the action endorsed herein.

This declaration is deemed fair and valid by both the American Bar Association and the Committee of Publishers Association and is legally binding throughout the United States.

Furthermore, the transmission, duplication or reproduction of any of the following work including specific information will be considered an illegal act irrespective of if it is done electronically or in print. This extends to creating a secondary or tertiary copy of the work or a recorded copy and is only allowed with express written consent from the Publisher. All additional right reserved.

The information in the following pages is broadly considered to be a truthful and accurate account of facts and as such any inattention, use or misuse of the information in question by the reader will render any resulting actions solely under their purview. There are no scenarios in which the publisher or the original author of this work can be in any fashion deemed liable for any hardship or damages that may befall them after undertaking information described herein.

Additionally, the information in the following pages is intended only for informational purposes and should thus be thought of as universal. As befitting its nature, it is presented without assurance regarding its prolonged validity or interim quality. Trademarks that are mentioned are done without written consent and can in no way be considered an endorsement from the trademark holder.

Table of Contents

PART I 11

    Grilling Rub 12

Chapter 1: Seafood 14

    Lemony Shrimp & Tomatoes 14

    Sea Bass With Garlic Butter 16

Chapter 2: Pork 18

    Grilled Sausages With Summer Veggies 18

    Honey-Chipotle Ribs 20

    Peachy Pork Ribs 22

    Pork Loin Steaks 24

Chapter 3: Poultry 26

    Chicago-Style Turkey Dogs 26

    Dr. Pepper Drumsticks 27

    Grilled Lemon Chicken 28

    Ground Turkey Burgers 30

    Spiced Chicken With Cilantro Lime Butter 32

    Turkey Pepper Kabobs 34

Chapter 4: Beef 35

    Classic Beef Cheeseburgers 36

    Grilled Skirt Steak With Peppers & Onions 38

    Tangy Lime Top Round Steak 40

    Whiskey Cheddar Burgers 42

Chapter 5: Dessert 44

Grilled Pineapple With Lime Dip 44

Take Care Of Your Grill! 46

PART II 47

Carnivore Diet 48

Chapter 1: What Is Carnivore Diet? 48

Chapter 2: Recipes for Tasty Appetizers 52

Oven-Baked Chicken Wings 52

Steak Nuggets 54

Grilled Shrimp 56

Roasted Bone Marrow 58

Bacon-Wrapped Chicken Bites 59

Salami Egg Muffins 60

3-Ingredients Scotch Eggs 61

Chapter 3: Quick and Easy Everyday Recipes 62

Carnivore Waffles 62

Chicken Bacon Pancakes 63

Garlic Cilantro Salmon 64

Mustard-Seared Bacon Burgers 66

Crockpot Shredded Chicken 68

Chapter 4: Weekend Dinner Recipes 69

Organ Meat Pie 69

Smokey Bacon Meatballs 70

Steak au Poivre 71

Skillet Rib Eye Steaks 73

Pan-Fried Pork Tenderloin 74

Carnivore Chicken Enchiladas 75

PART III 77

Chapter 1: Soup 78

    Hot & Sour Soup 78

    Wonton Soup 80

Chapter 2: Seafood 81

    Honey Walnut Shrimp 81

    Steamed Fish 83

    Stir-Fried Shrimp & Scallions 85

Chapter 3: Poultry 86

    Kung Pao Chicken - Keto-Friendly 87

    Orange Chicken 90

Chapter 4: Pork 92

    Chinese Pork BBQ (Char Siu) 92

    Chinese Pork Dumplings 94

    Chop Suey 95

    Easy Moo Shu Pork 97

    Peking Pork Chops - Slow-Cooked 98

Chapter 5: Other Chinese Dishes 100

    Crispy Tofu With Sweet & Sour Sauce 100

    Shiitake & Scallion Lo Mein 102

PART IV 104

Chapter 1: Tasty Breakfast Options 105

    French Crepe 105

Chapter 2: Delicious Salads 109

    Traditional French Country Salad With Lemon Dijon Vinaigrette 109

Chapter 3: Soup 111

Classic French Onion Bistro Soup 111

Fresh French Pea Soup 113

Green Vegetable Soup 115

Chapter 4: Beef Options **117**

Beef Bourguignon - Slow-Cooked 117

Entrecote Steak With Red Wine Sauce 119

Pan-Seared Steak au Poivre 121

Steak Diane 123

Chapter 5: Other Delicious French Classics **125**

French Ham & Grilled Cheese Sandwich - Croque Monsieur 125

Pork Chops With Mustard Sauce 127

Provencal Chicken Casserole 129

White Wine Coq Au Vin 130

PART V **132**

Chapter 1: Health Benefits of the Hormone Diet 133

Chapter 2: Hormone-Rebalancing Smoothies 136

    Estrogen Detox Smoothie 136

    Dopamine Delight Smoothie 138

    Breakfast Smoothie Bowl 139

    Blueberry Detox Smoothie 141

    Maca Mango Smoothie 142

    Pituitary Relief Smoothie 143

Chapter 2: Easy Breakfast Recipes 144

    Scrambled Eggs With Feta and Tomatoes 144

    Smashed Avo and Quinoa 146

    Hormone Balancing Granola 148

Chapter 3: Healthy Lunch Recipes 150
- Easy Shakshuka 150
- Ginger Chicken 152
- Carrot and Miso Soup 154
- Arugula Salad 156
- Kale Soup 158
- Roasted Sardines 159

Chapter 4: Tasty Dinner Recipes 161
- Rosemary Chicken 162
- Corned Beef and Cabbage 163
- Roasted Parsnips and Carrots 164
- Herbed Salmon 165
- Chipotle Cauliflower Tacos 167

PART VI 169

Chapter 1: What is The Freestyle Way? 170
- Zero Point Fruits 171
- Zero Point Vegetables 171
- Zero Point Spices & Other Condiments 171
- Other Foods To Enjoy Freestyle 172

Chapter 2: Breakfast Favourites 173
- Baked Omelet 173
- Banana Roll-Ups 174
- Broccoli Cheddar Egg Muffins 175
- Cinnamon-Apple French Toast 176
- Country Cottage Pancakes 177
- Egg & Sausage Muffins 178

Egg &Veggie Scramble 179

Hard-Boiled Eggs in the Instant Pot 180

Muffin Tin Eggs 181

Tropical Breakfast Pie 182

Chapter 3: lunch favorites 185

Chapter 4: scrumptious dinner choices: Beef – Fish & Seafood 198

Chapter 5: scrumptious dinner choices: Pork & poultry 205

Chapter 6: Delicious sides 213

Chapter 7: 21-day meal plan 221

PART I

Before we get started on your new recipes, let's learn how to make a delicious rub for your favorite meat.

Grilling Rub

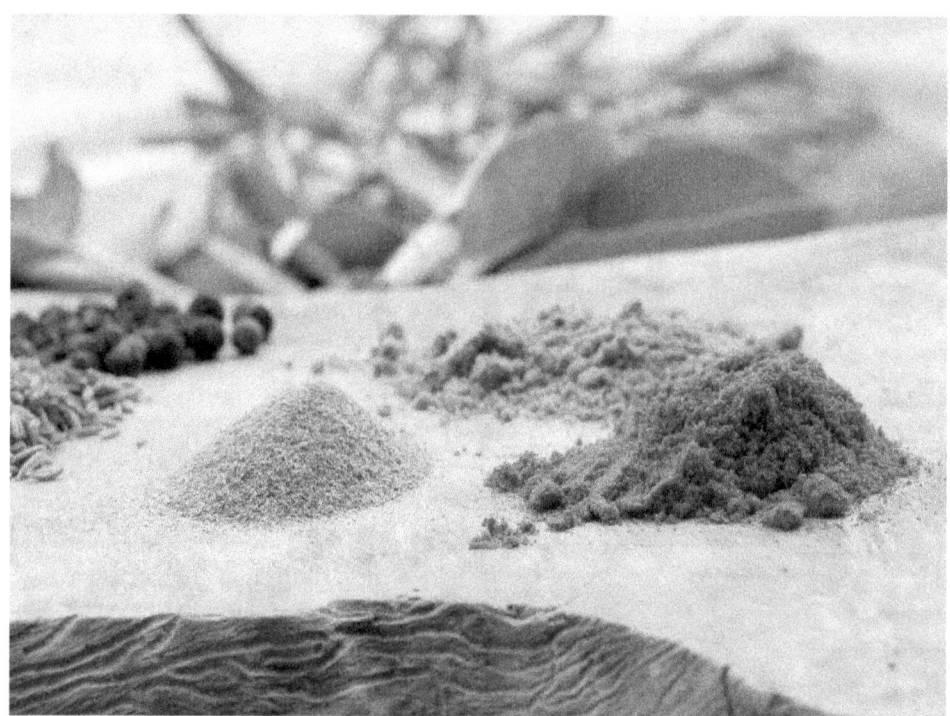

What is Needed:

- Finely ground dark-roast coffee (3 tbsp.)
- Chili powder (3 tbsp.)
- Chipotle powder (1 tsp.)
- Dark brown sugar (3 tbsp.)
- Kosher salt (2 tbsp.)

- Smoked paprika (2 tbsp.)
- Dried thyme (1 tbsp.)
- Granulated garlic (1 tbsp.)
- Ground cumin (2 tsp.)

Preparation Method:

1. Be sure to pack the sugar when it's measured - tightly. Combine each of the fixings and rub them into the chosen meat.
2. Leave the rub on the meat for 12-24 hours before grilling.

Chapter 1: Seafood

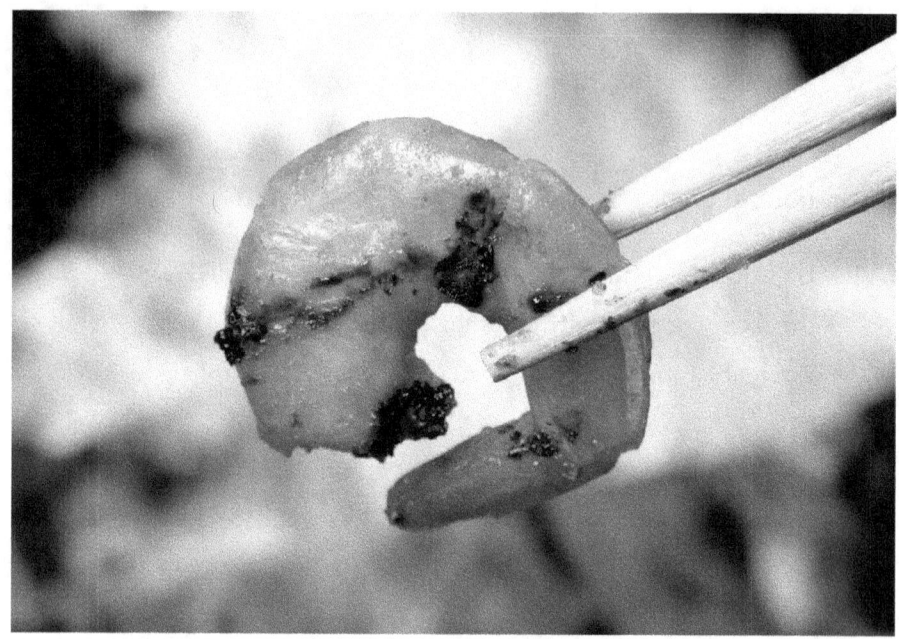

Lemony Shrimp & Tomatoes

Servings Provided: 4 kabobs with ½ cup sauce each

Time Required: 25 minutes

What is Needed:

- Olive oil (2 tbsp.)
- Lemon juice (.33 cup)
- Grated lemon zest (.5 tsp.)
- Uncooked jumbo shrimp (1 lb.)
- Fresh arugula (2/3 cup)

- Sliced green onions (2)
- Plain yogurt (.25 cup)
- 2% milk (2 tsp.)
- Cider vinegar (1 tsp.)
- Sugar (.5 tsp.)
- Garlic (2 cloves)
- Dijon mustard (1 tsp.)
- Salt (.5 tsp. divided)
- Cherry tomatoes (12)
- Pepper (.25 tsp.)
- Also Needed: Skewers (4)

Preparation Method:

1. If you plan to use wooden skewers, be sure to soak them in water before you thread them.
2. Prepare a large mixing container and add the lemon juice, oil, minced garlic, and lemon zest, whisking until blended.
3. Fold in the shrimp and wait for about ten minutes.
4. Rinse and toss the arugula, green onions, yogurt, milk, vinegar, mustard, sugar, and ¼ of teaspoon salt in a food processor, pulsing until smooth.
5. Peel and devein the shrimp.
6. Prepare the skewers by alternating using the shrimp and tomatoes. Sprinkle it with pepper and rest of the salt.
7. Grill, covered, using the med-high temperature setting for two to three minutes per side or until shrimp are no longer pink.
8. Serve the kabobs with sauce.

Sea Bass With Garlic Butter

Servings Provided: 4

Time Required: 25 minutes

What is Needed:

- Sea bass (2 lb.)
- Butter (3 tbsp.)
- Lemon juice (1 medium lemon)
- Italian parsley (2 tbsp.)
- Olive oil (1.5 tbsp.)
- Cloves of garlic (2)

   Spices - .25 tsp. each:

- Garlic powder
- Paprika
- Onion powder
- Sea salt

Preparation Method:

1. Mince the garlic and finely chop the parsley.
2. Make the sauce. Prepare a saucepan to melt the butter and combine it with the lemon juice, garlic, and parsley. Transfer the pan to a cool burner once the butter has melted.
3. Warm the grill using the med-high temperature setting.

4. Oil the grates right before placing the fish onto the grill.
5. Combine the garlic, onion powder, paprika, pepper, and salt in a small mixing bowl.
6. Sprinkle the seasoning mixture on each side of the fish.
7. Grill the sea bass for seven minutes. Turn the fish and coat it with the butter sauce. Grill it for about seven additional minutes.
8. Once the fish reaches an internal temperature of at least 145° Fahrenheit, remove it from the heat, and spritz it with olive oil.
9. Serve it with your favorite sides.

Chapter 2: Pork

Grilled Sausages With Summer Veggies

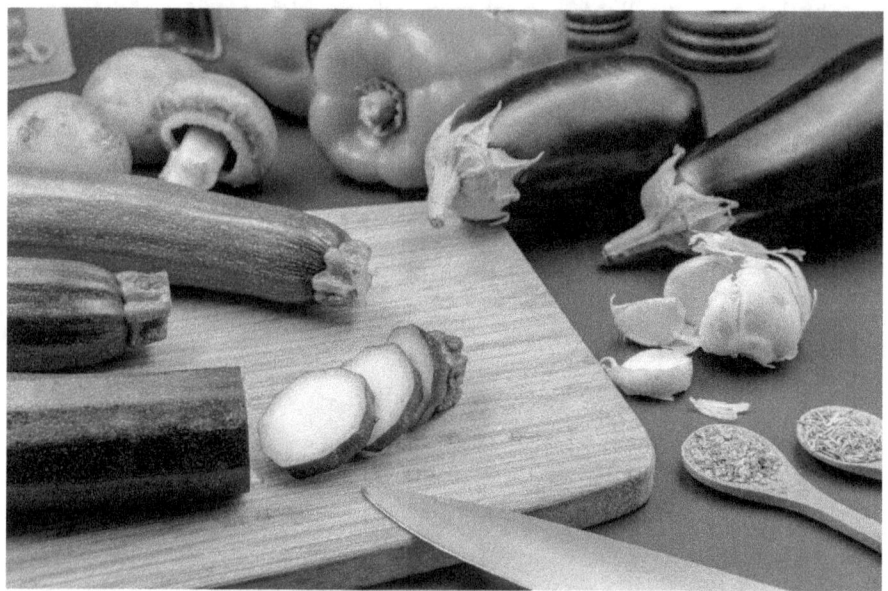

Servings Provided: 12

Time Required: 60 minutes

What is Needed:

- Peach preserves (.75 cup)
- Soy sauce (.5 cup)
- Freshly minced ginger root (.5 cup)
- Water (3 tbsp.)
- Garlic (3 minced cloves)

- Optional: Hot pepper sauce (1 dash)
- Sweet red peppers (4 medium)
- Zucchini (3 small)
- Eggplant (1 medium)
- Yellow summer squash (2 small)
- Italian pork/turkey sausage links (12 hot @ 4 oz. each)

Preparation Method:

1. Measure and add the first five ingredients (up to the line) in a blender, adding the pepper sauce as desired. Cover with the lid and mix until blended.
2. Slice the zucchini and yellow squash lengthwise into quarters. Slice the peppers lengthwise in half and remove the seeds. Cut eggplant lengthwise into 1/2-inch-thick slices. Place all vegetables in a big mixing container and drizzle them using ½ cup of the sauce and toss to coat.
3. Place the veggies onto a greased grill rack. Grill, covered using medium heat until tender and lightly charred, turning once (8-10 min.). Cool slightly and adjust the grill temperature to the med-low setting.
4. Cut vegetables into bite-sized pieces. Toss with an additional ¼ cup sauce and keep warm.
5. Grill the sausages, covered, on med-low heat setting for 15-20 minutes or until a thermometer reads 160° Fahrenheit for pork sausages (165° Fahrenheit for turkey sausages) - turning occasionally. Remove sausages from grill and toss with the remaining sauce. Serve with vegetables.

Honey-Chipotle Ribs

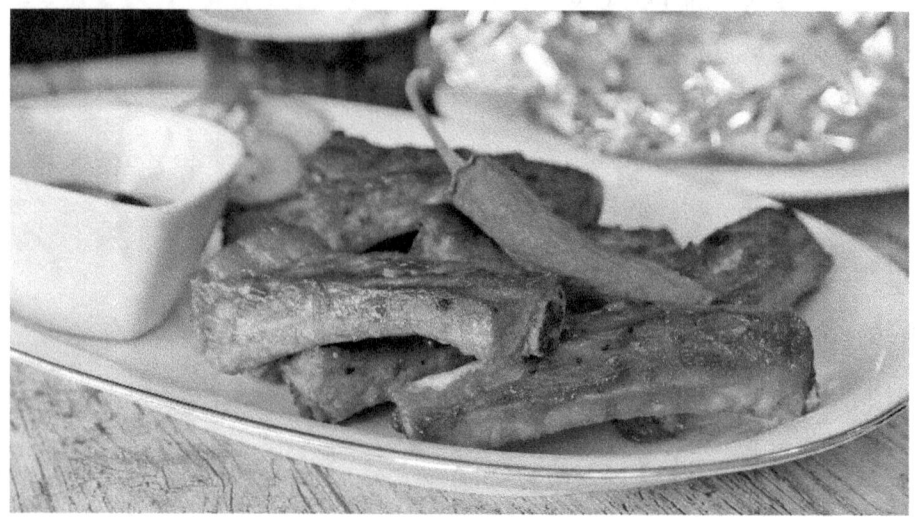

Servings Provided: 12

Time Required: 1 hour 35 minutes

What is Needed:

- Pork baby back ribs (6 lb.)
  The Sauce:

- Ground chipotle pepper (4 tsp.)
- Chipotle peppers - in adobo sauce (2 tbsp.)
- Guinness beer (2 bottles - 11.2 oz ea.)
- Ketchup (3 cups)
- BBQ sauce (2 cups)

- Honey (2/3 cup)
- Onion (1 small)
- Worcestershire sauce (.25 cup)
- Dijon mustard (2 tbsp.)
- Black pepper (.5 tsp.)
- Salt (1 tsp.)
- Garlic powder (1 tsp.)

Preparation Method:

1. Chop the onion and chipotle peppers.
2. Wrap the ribs in large pieces of heavy-duty foil, sealing the edges of foil.
3. Grill the ribs with the lid 'on' while using indirect medium heat until tender (1-1.5 hrs.).
4. Combine the sauce ingredients in a large saucepan.
5. Adjust the temperature setting to simmer, uncovered, for about 45 minutes - until thickened - stirring occasionally.
6. Remove ribs from foil and place over direct heat. Baste them with some of the sauce.
7. Grill the ribs with the lid on, using the medium temperature setting for about half an hour or until browned, turning once and occasionally basting with additional sauce.
8. Serve with the rest of the sauce.

Peachy Pork Ribs

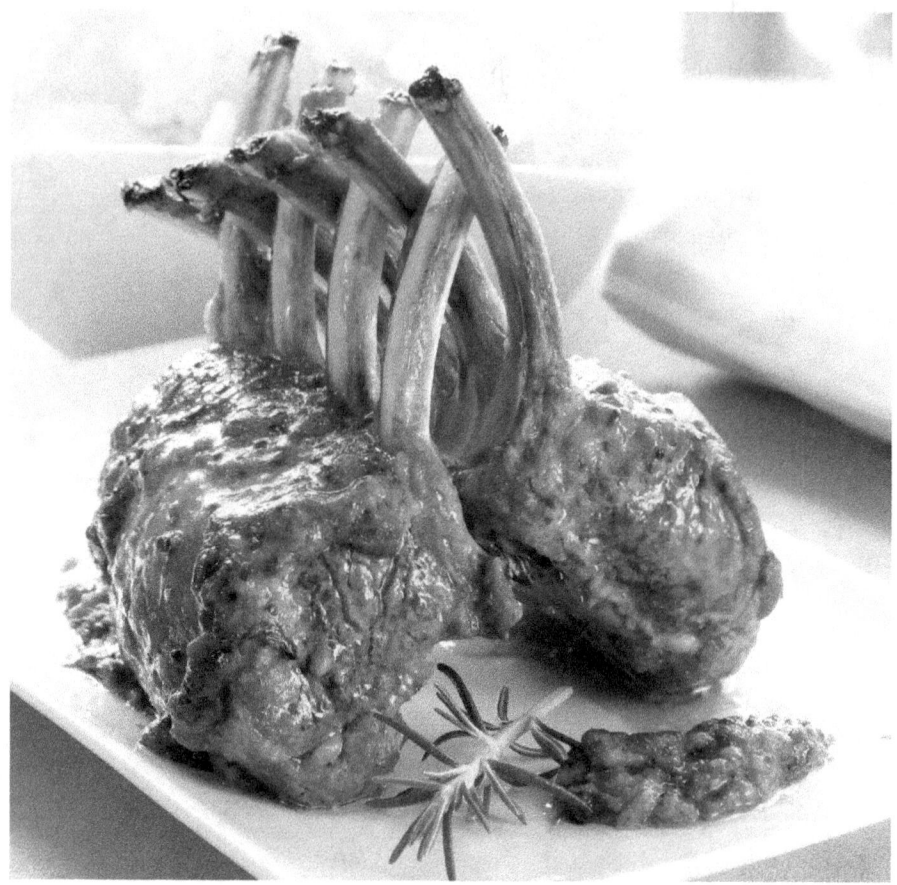

Servings Provided: 4

Time Required: 2.5 hours

What is Needed:

- Pork baby back ribs (4 lb./in serving-sized portions)

- Water (.5 cup)
- Ripe peaches (3 medium)
- Onion (2 tbsp.)
- Butter (2 tbsp.)
- Garlic (1 clove)
- Lemon juice (3 tbsp.)
- Orange juice concentrate (2 tbsp.)
- Soy sauce (2 tsp.)
- Ground mustard (.5 tsp.)
- Brown sugar (1 tbsp.)
- Salt (.25 tsp.)

Preparation Method:

1. Mince the garlic and onion.
2. Add the ribs into a shallow roasting pan of water.
3. Place a layer of foil over the pan, and bake at 325° Fahrenheit for two hours.
4. Peel and cube the peaches and toss them into a blender, cover, and process until blended.
5. Prepare a small saucepan to melt the butter. Sauté the onion until tender. Mix in the garlic and sauté for one more minute. Stir in the lemon juice, orange juice concentrate, soy sauce, brown sugar, mustard, pepper, salt, and pureed peaches. Warm until thoroughly heated.
6. Drain the ribs. Spoon some of the sauce over ribs.
7. Grill the ribs using the medium temperature setting on a lightly oiled rack, covered, for eight to ten minutes or until browned, turning occasionally and brushing with sauce.

Pork Loin Steaks

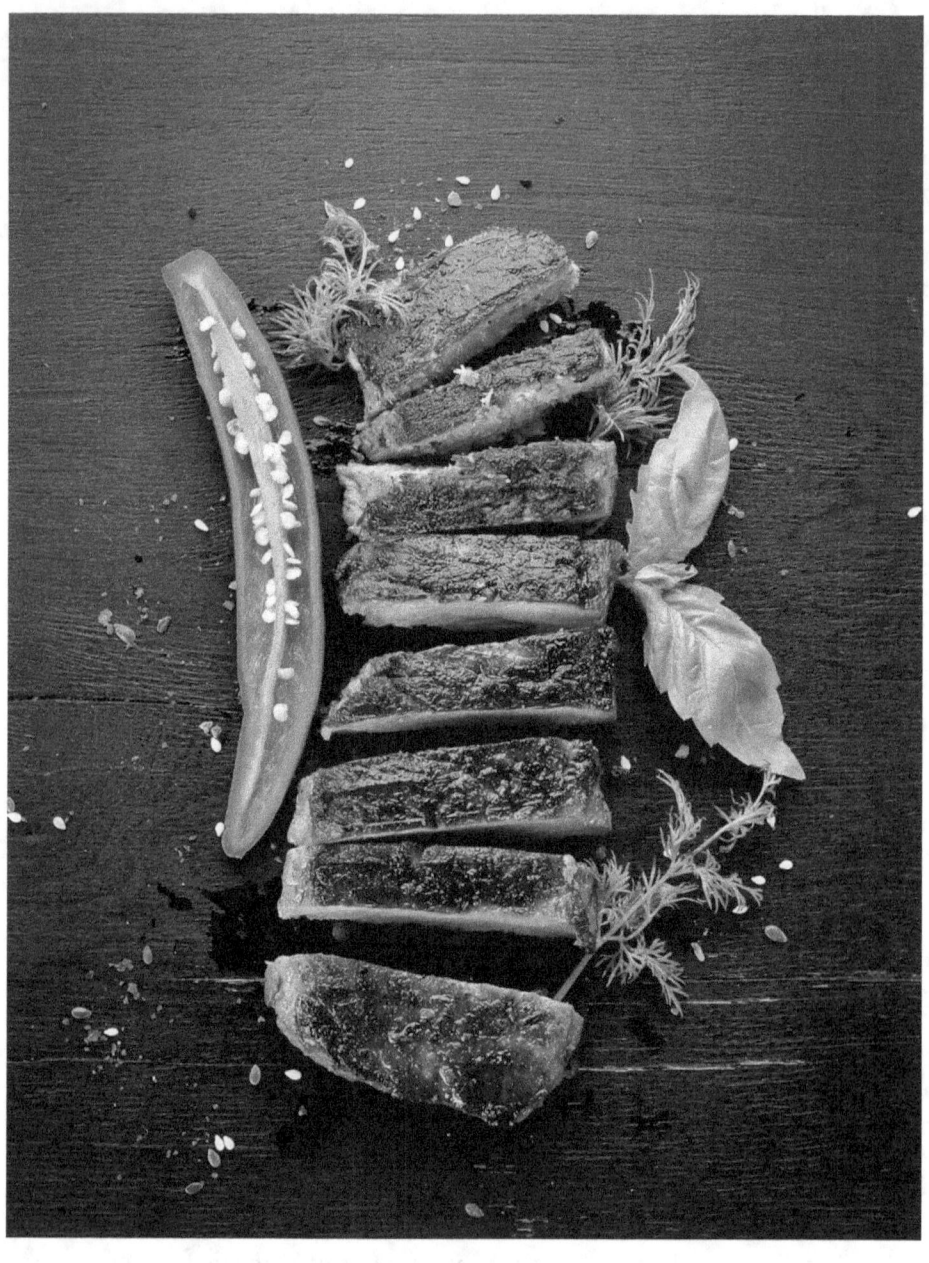

Servings Provided: 2

Time Required: 25 minutes

What is Needed:

- Pork loin steaks (4 boneless)
- Water (.25 cup)
- Dried oregano (1 tsp.)
- Brown sugar (2 tbsp.)

Preparation Method:

1. Use a non-metallic container to combine the marinade fixings.
2. Add the steaks to the bowl and cover to marinate overnight or for a minimum of two hours in the fridge.
3. Prepare the grill using the med-high temperature setting.
4. Grill the steaks for three to five minutes on each side and serve with your favorite side dishes.

Chapter 3: Poultry

Chicago-Style Turkey Dogs

Servings Provided: 4

Time Required: 20 minutes

What is Needed:

- Turkey hot dogs (4)
- Whole wheat tortillas (4 @ 8-inch - warmed)
- Sandwich pickle slices (4 thin)
- Chopped sweet onions (.5 cup)
- Optional Toppings:
- Prepared mustard
- Pickled hot peppers
- Cheddar cheese

Preparation Method:

1. Grill the hot dogs until they are as you like them - with the grill marks.
2. Serve in a tortilla with a portion of tomatoes, cucumber, pickles, and onions.
3. Add more toppings as desired.

Dr. Pepper Drumsticks

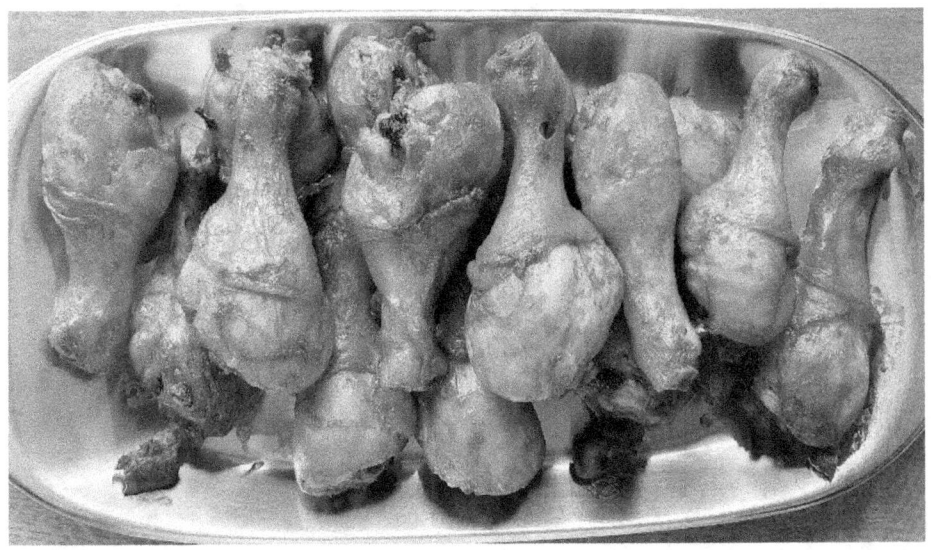

Servings Provided: 6

Time Required: 50 minutes

What is Needed:

- Dr. Pepper (2/3 cup)
- Ketchup (1 cup)
- Bourbon (2 tbsp.)
- Brown sugar (2 tbsp.)
- Salt (.125 tsp.)
- BBQ seasoning (4 tsp.)
- Worcestershire sauce (1 tbsp.)
- Optional: Celery salt (.25 tsp.)
- Chicken drumsticks (12)

Preparation Method:

1. Combine the sauce fixings (up to the line) in a saucepan. Add the celery salt as desired. Wait for it to boil and adjust the temperature setting to simmer, uncovered, for eight to ten minutes or until slightly thickened, stirring often.
2. On an oiled grill using the med-low temperature setting, cook the chicken, covered for 15 minutes. Turn and continue to grill 15-20 minutes until an internal thermometer reads 170°-175° Fahrenheit. Brush it occasionally with sauce.

Grilled Lemon Chicken

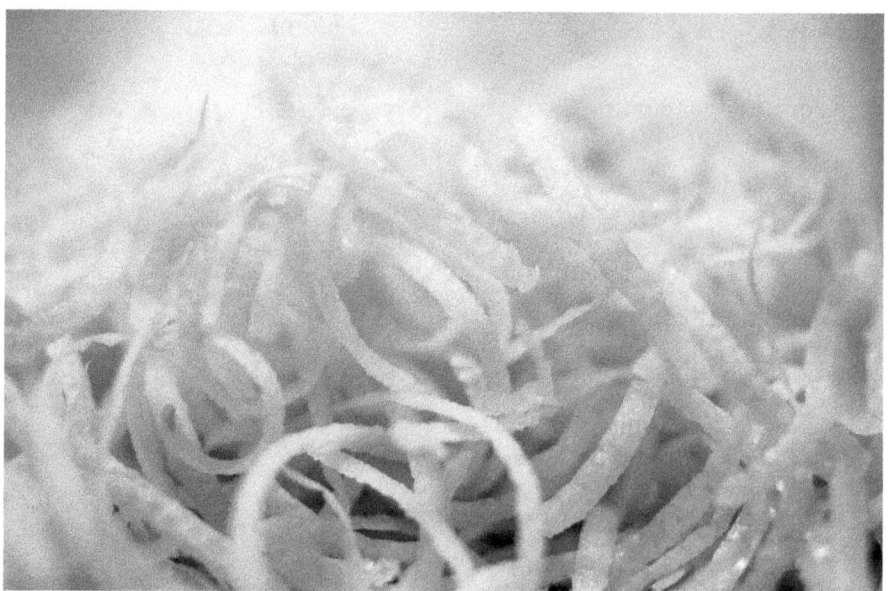

Servings Provided: 12

Time Required: 45 minutes

What is Needed:

- Fryer/broiler chickens - cut up (3-3.5 lb. each)
- Lemonade concentrate - thawed (.75 cup)
- Soy sauce (.33 cup)
- Garlic (1 clove)
- Seasoned salt (1 tsp.)
- Garlic powder (.125 tsp.)
- Celery salt (.5 tsp.)

Preparation Method:

1. Mince the garlic and mix all of the fixings except for the pieces of chicken.
2. Pour half of the mixture into a shallow glass dish. Use a layer of foil or plastic to cover the bowl and place the rest of the lemonade mixture in the fridge.
3. Dip the chicken into lemonade mixture, turning to coat and trash the used marinade.
4. Grill the chicken, covered, using the medium-temperature setting for 30 minutes, turning occasionally. Brush with the reserved lemonade mixture.
5. Grill it for another 10-20 minutes, frequently basting, until a thermometer reads 165° Fahrenheit.

Ground Turkey Burgers

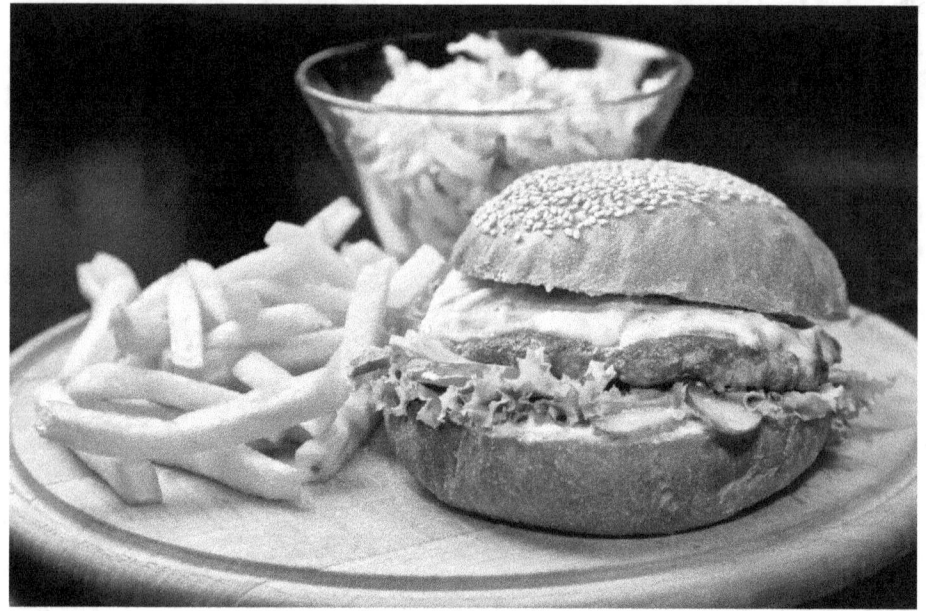

Servings Provided: 6

Time Required: 30 minutes

What is Needed:

- Whisked egg (1 large)
- Whole wheat breadcrumbs (2/3 cup)
- Celery (.5 cup)
- Onion (.25 cup)
- Freshly minced parsley (1 tbsp.)
- Worcestershire sauce (1 tsp.)

- Pepper (.25 tsp)
- Salt (.5 tsp.)
- Dried oregano (1 tsp.)
- Lean ground turkey (1.25 lb.)
- Split whole wheat burger buns (6 whole)

Preparation Method:

1. Chop the onion and celery.
2. Combine the breadcrumbs, egg, celery, seasonings, onion, parsley, and Worcestershire sauce.
3. Add the turkey and shape into patties.
4. Prepare on the grill using the medium-temperature setting until they reach an internal temp of 165° Fahrenheit.
5. Serve the burgers on the buns as desired.

Spiced Chicken With Cilantro Lime Butter

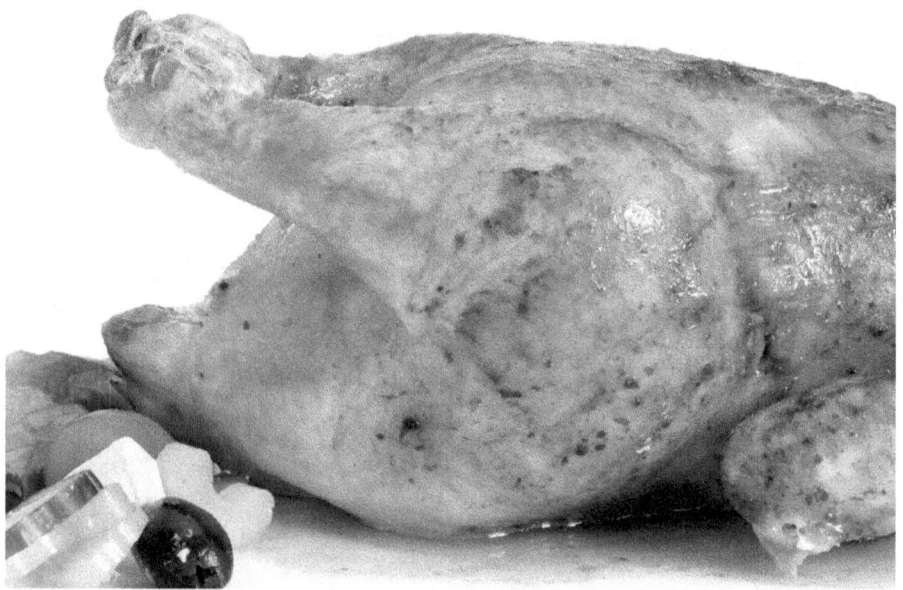

Servings Provided: 6

Time Required: 55 minutes

What is Needed:

The Sauce Ingredients:

- Chili powder (1 tbsp.)
- Ground cinnamon (2 tsp.)
- Brown sugar (1 tbsp.)
- Baking cocoa (1 tsp.)
- Balsamic vinegar (1 tbsp.)
- Pepper & salt (.5 tsp. each)
- Olive oil (3 tbsp.)
- Bone-in breast halves (6 @ 8 oz. each)

The Lime Butter:

- Melted butter (.33 cup)
- Cilantro (.25 cup)
- Red onion (2 tbsp.)
- Serrano pepper (1)
- Black pepper (.125 tsp.)
- Lime juice (1 tbsp.)

Preparation Method:

1. Finely chop the cilantro, onion, and serrano pepper.
2. Combine the sauce fixings; brown sugar, chili powder, cinnamon, cocoa, pepper, salt, vinegar, and oil. Brush the mixture over chicken.
3. Arrange the chicken skin-side down on the grill rack.
4. Grill the chicken - covered for 15 minutes (indirect medium heat).
5. Flip it over and continue to grill for 20-25 minutes longer (internal temp of 165 °Fahrenheit.
6. Combine the butter fixings to drizzle over the chicken before serving.

Turkey Pepper Kabobs

Servings Provided: 4

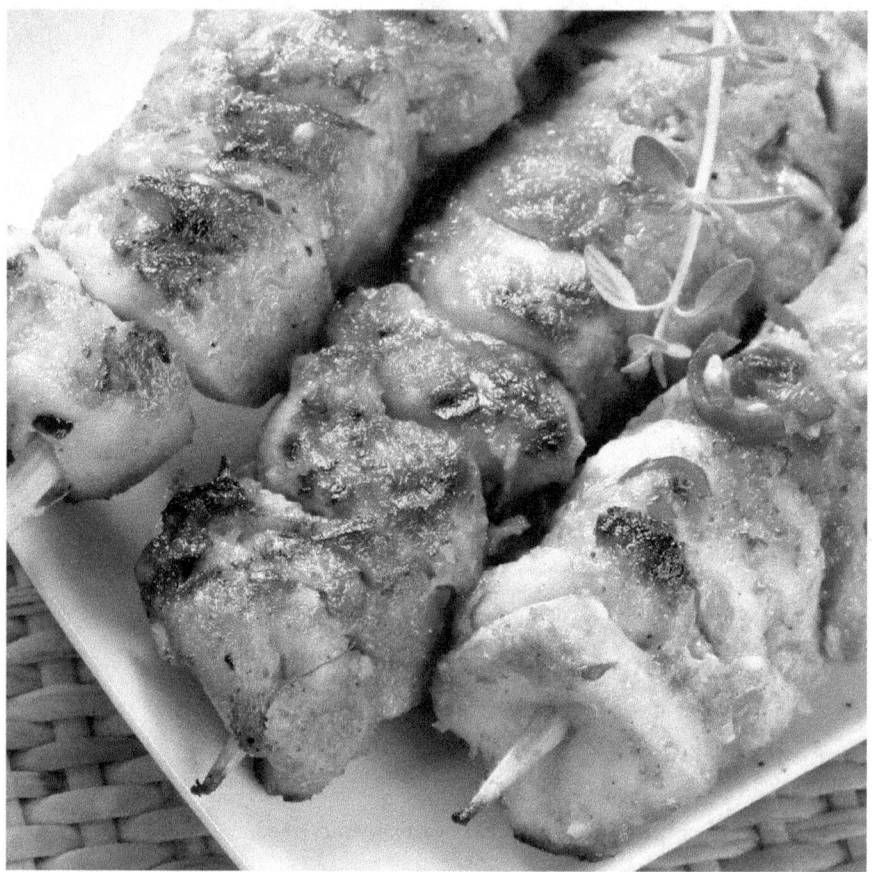

Time Required: 25 minutes

What is Needed:

- Unsweetened pineapple chunks (8 oz. can)
- Brown sugar (.25 cup - packed)

- Worcestershire sauce (2 tbsp.)
- Canola oil (2 tbsp.)
- Garlic (1 clove)
- Prepared mustard (1 tsp.)
- Turkey breast tenderloins (1 lb.)
- Green pepper (1 large)
- Sweet onion (1 large - 0.75-inch pieces)
- Red sweet pepper (1 large)

Preparation Method:

1. Chop the turkey and sweet peppers into one-inch pieces.
2. Drain the pineapple, saving ¼ cup of the juice.
3. Prepare the marinade by mixing the brown sugar with the oil, mustard, Worcestershire sauce, minced garlic, and reserved juice.
4. In another mixing container, cube and toss in the turkey with 1/3 cup of marinade. Refrigerate it covered for two to three hours. Cover and refrigerate the rest of the marinade.
5. On eight soaked wooden skewers or metal, alternately thread the turkey, veggies, and pineapple chunks. Discard the remaining marinade.
6. Arrange the kabobs on an oiled grill rack using medium heat. Grill, covered, until the turkey is no longer pink (8-10 min.), turning occasionally
7. Note: Baste them frequently with the reserved marinade during the last three minutes.

Chapter 4: Beef

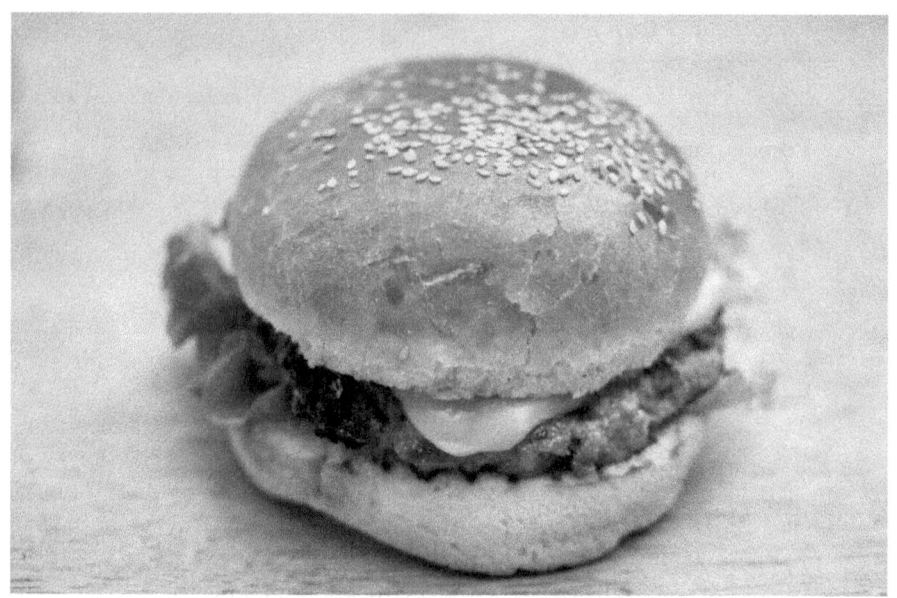

Classic Beef Cheeseburgers

Servings Provided: 4

Time Required: 30 minutes

What is Needed:

- 90% lean ground beef (1 lb.)
- Steak seasoning blend (1.5 tsp.)
- Burger buns (4 - split)
- American/Cheddar/Swiss cheese (4 slices)
- Lettuce (4 leaves)
- Tomato (4 slices)

Optional Toppings:

- Mustard
- Ketchup
- Onion slices
- Pickle slices

Preparation Method:

1. Prepare the grill until it reaches medium ash-covered coals.
2. While it heats, mix the beef and steak seasoning in a large mixing container, shaping it into four ½ -inch thick patties.
3. Arrange the patties on the grid over the coals. Grill the burgers covered for 8 to 10 minutes (for a gas grill 7-9 min.), occasionally turning until an instant-read thermometer inserted horizontally into its center registers at 160° Fahrenheit.
4. About two minutes before the burgers are done, arrange the buns, cut side down, on the grid. Grill until lightly toasted. During the last minute of grilling, top each burger with a slice of cheese to melt.
5. Line the bottom of each bun with lettuce, topping it with the burger, tomato, and chosen toppings. Close the sandwiches and serve.

Grilled Skirt Steak With Peppers & Onions

Servings Provided: 6

Time Required: 50 minutes

What is Needed:

- Apple juice (.5 cup)
- Red wine vinegar (.5 cup)
- Yellow/white onion (.25 cup)
- Rubbed sage (2 tbsp.)
- Ground mustard (3 tsp.)
- Salt (1 tsp.)
- Ground coriander (3 tsp.)
- Black pepper (3 tsp.)
- Garlic clove (1 minced)
- Olive oil (1 cup)
- Beef skirt steak (1.5 lb.)
- Red onions (2 medium)
- Sweet red peppers (2 medium)
- Green onions (12)

Preparation Method:

1. Finely chop the onion, slice the peppers into halves, and trim the green onions. Cut the steak into 5-inch pieces and slice the red onions into ½-in slices.
2. Whisk the first nine ingredients (up to the line) until blended.
3. Slowly whisk in oil. Pour 1.5 cups of the marinade into a large resealable plastic bag. Toss in the beef and seal the bag - tossing it to coat. Refrigerate it overnight. Also, cover and refrigerate the rest of the marinade.
4. Toss the rest of the veggies with ¼ cup of the reserved marinade. Grill the red onions and peppers, covered, using the medium temperature setting (4-6 min. per side)until tender. Grill the green onions one to two minutes until tender.
5. Drain the beef, and trash the marinade in the bag.
6. Grill the beef covered using medium heat (4-6 min. per side) until the meat reaches desired doneness (for medium-rare, a thermometer should read 135° Fahrenheit; medium, 140° Fahrenheit; medium-well, 145° Fahrenheit). Baste with the remaining marinade during the last four minutes of cooking. Let the steak stand for five minutes.
7. Chop the veggies into small pieces and transfer them into an over-sized mixing container. Slice the steak diagonally across the grain into thin slices, add to vegetables, and toss to combine.
8. Serve and enjoy it when it's ready.

Tangy Lime Top Round Steak

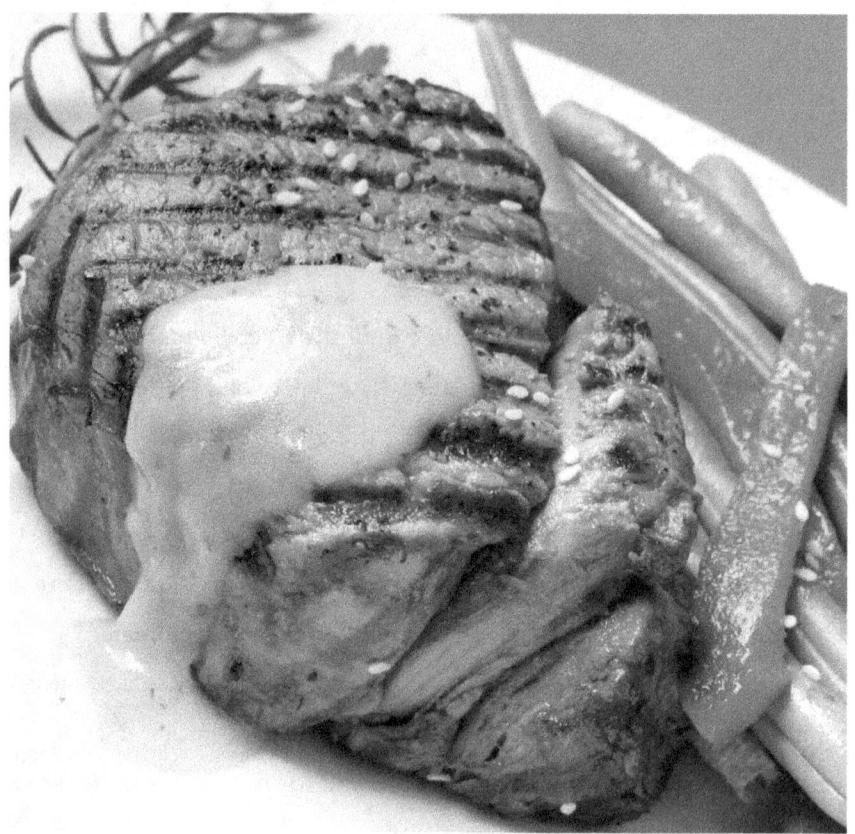

Servings Provided: 4

Time Required: 25 minutes

What is Needed:

- Top round steak (1 lb.)
- Fresh lime juice (.25 cup)
- Worcestershire sauce (1 tbsp.)
- Brown sugar - lightly packed (2 tbsp.)
- Vegetable oil (2 tbsp.)

- Garlic (1 tbsp. - minced)

Preparation Method:

1. Whisk the juice, sugar, oil, Worcestershire, and minced garlic in a small mixing container.
2. Trim the steak, slicing it to a ¾-inch thickness.
3. Place the steak and lime mixture in a zipper-type plastic bag; toss the steak to coat. Securely close the bag and marinate in the fridge for six hours or overnight - turning intermittently.
4. Trash the marinade and place the steak on the grill grid using medium ash-covered coals.
5. Grill, covered for 10-11 minutes, turning occasionally. Don't overcook it. (For medium-rare: 145° Fahrenheit internal temp.)
6. Carve the steak into thin slices.

Whiskey Cheddar Burgers

Servings Provided: 8

Time Required: 30 minutes

What is Needed:

- Whiskey (.25 cup)

- Soy sauce (1 tbsp.)

- Black pepper and salt (.5 tsp. each)

- Worcestershire sauce (1 tbsp.)

- Shredded sharp cheddar cheese (1 cup)

- Onion (.25 cup)

- Seasoned breadcrumbs (2 tbsp.)

- Cloves of garlic (3)

- Paprika (.5 tsp.)

- Dried basil (.5 tsp.)

- Lean ground beef (1.5 lb.)

- Onion/burger buns - split (8)

    Optional Toppings:

- Lettuce
- Sliced tomatoes
- BBQ sauce
- Cheddar cheese slice

Preparation Method:

1. Finely chop the onions and cloves. Combine all of the fixings, adding the beef, last.
2. Thoroughly, but gently, combine the mix shaping it into eight ½-inch-thick patties.
3. Prepare a greased grill, using the medium temperature setting.
4. Cook the burgers, covered, for four to five minutes on each side or until a thermometer reads 160° Fahrenheit (internally).
5. Serve the burgers on rolls with toppings as desired.

Chapter 5: Dessert

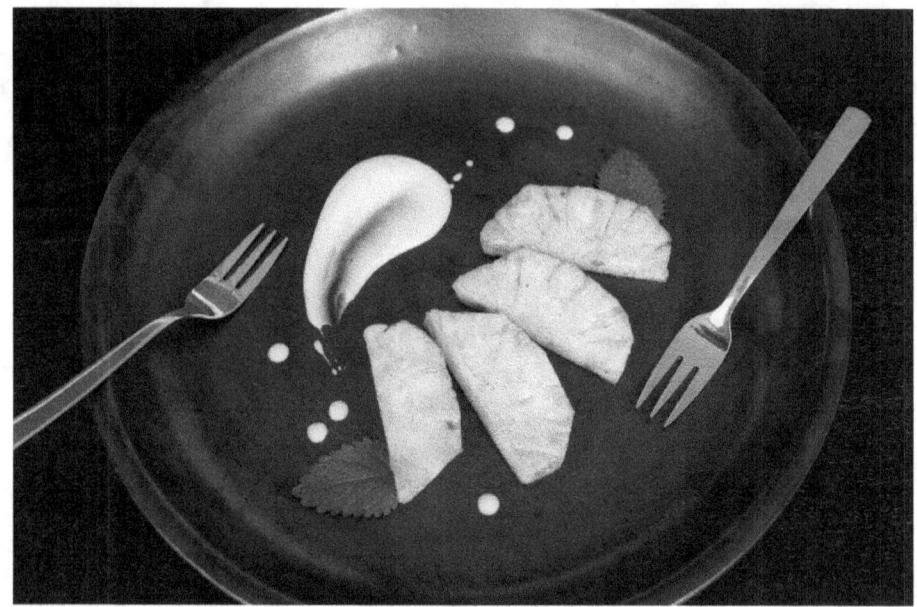

Grilled Pineapple With Lime Dip

Servings Provided: 8

Time Required: 30 minutes

What is Needed:

- Fresh pineapple (1)
- Lime juice (2 tbsp.)
- Packed brown sugar (.25 cup)
- Honey (3 tbsp.)

The Dip:

- Grated lime zest (1 tsp.)
- Brown sugar (1 tbsp.)
- Lime juice (1 tbsp.)
- Honey (2 tbsp.)
- Unchilled cream cheese (3 oz.)
- Plain yogurt (.25 cup)

Preparation Method:

1. Spritz the grill rack using a cooking oil spray before warming the grill. Peel and core the pineapple and slice it vertically into eight wedges. Cut each wedge horizontally into two spears.
2. Combine the honey, brown sugar, and lime juice in a shallow dish and add the pineapple. Toss it and cover to refrigerate for one hour.
3. Beat cream cheese until smooth. Mix in the yogurt with the honey, brown sugar, lime juice, and zest. Cover and pop it into the fridge until it's time to serve.
4. Drain the pineapple, discarding marinade. Grill the pineapple spears using the medium temperature setting (lid on) for three to four minutes per side or until they have grill marks that are golden brown. Serve with the lime dip.

Take Care Of Your Grill!

How to Clean the Grill:

1. Gather a few folded paper towels. Use a large pair of tongs and a high smoke point oil (ex. peanut, sunflower, canola). Olive oil will work in a pinch.
2. Dip the paper towels into a portion of the chosen oil and run it across the grates at least three times to create a non-stick surface to help prevent the meat or fish from breaking during the cooking process.
3. Easy - yet healthy!

PART II

Carnivore Diet

For all the meat lovers out there, the next diet that we are going to discuss is known as the carnivore diet.

Chapter 1: What Is Carnivore Diet?

The Carnivore Diet is the all-new trendy diet that expects its followers to go on a meat-only way of lifestyle. This diet completely goes against nutritional stereotyping. If someone asked you to replace that bowl of meat with vegetable oils and carbs, you probably have been misled!

This diet has won favor for several reasons and is, of course, not a fluke. If you find it attractive to sink in a carnivore way of eating, you have come to the right place.

The carnivore diet is the one that entirely revolves around a meat-based pattern of eating. It is one extreme diet that restricts you from eating plant-based foods and strictly opposes carbohydrate consumption. It might sound crazy, but there are people including Shawn Baker (the creator of this diet) who have normalized this fact that carbohydrate is a non-essential macronutrient, and there is no harm in cutting them down from the menu.

It is a zero-carb diet that altogether emphasizes consuming meat. Scientists consider this diet the best nutrition source for human beings, cutting out the chatter from plant toxins.

Science Behind Carnivore Diet: Reasons Why This Diet Will Work

There are more anecdotes and testimonials than research backed up with science. This no-carb diet has also been a second option to those who have either failed to carry on with Paleo and Keto diet or have faced other severe consequences after following them. This is a bold claim and has a lot to unpack. Let's dive deep into the depth of its science.

Researchers have carried out several studies throughout the Earth that has proved its benefits on humankind.

- **Removes the Inflammatory Vegetables -** If you have been suffering from an autoimmune disorder or a damaged gut, this might be of concern.

    Almost every vegetable has some kind of toxin in it. Brussels Sprouts, broccoli, cauliflower have sulforaphane that causes hypothyroidism and damage to health. Nightshades damage carb and fat metabolism. Polyphenols cause DNA damage. Lectins cause leaky guts. Reservatrol can inhibit androgen precursors. Spinach has oxalates that may result in kidney stones, and the list goes on. Choosing a carnivore diet can be a game-changing plan for such people and others who are still being manipulated by conventional nutritional advice.

- **It Increases Cholesterol –** You all must have heard about bad and good cholesterol. Cholesterol plays a negative role when it is oxidized or damaged and gets trapped in the artery walls. LDL cholesterol, even though it is given the tag of the 'bad' cholesterol, protects your body from diseases and does not cause them. They bind to the pathogens allowing the immune system to expel them.

  During inflammation, the body uses LDL as a protective mechanism. So, people with heart diseases have high LDL levels because it binds to the pathogens, getting rid of the damage ensuring that it does not spread. It is, in fact, the inflammation that causes heart diseases.

- **It Increases the Nutrient Density** - Animal-based foods have the most bioavailable form of nutrients that play a crucial role from growth to brain function. While you have been a fiber-freak, you might just have missed out on the essential nutrients. Vegetarians have a deficiency in Vitamin B12 and Iron. Americans have Vitamin D deficiency, and women have Calcium deficiency, while Zinc is a deficient nutrient worldwide.

  The brain requires micronutrients, and it is animals that mostly provide this. Zinc and iron are vital nutrients that help brain growth, dopamine transport, and serotonin synthesis.

- **It Reverses Insulin Resistance -** The best thing you could do to your health is reverse the insulin resistance. It is a problem where your body's cells become unresponsive to insulin action and therefore refuse to stuff the cells with more energy, leading to a rise in insulin level. It occurs due to excess carbohydrates and fat that shut off the process of burning fat, causing the fat to be stored without being used directly. The carnivore diet can be a solution to this!

- **Weight loss** - Since protein-based foods are satiating, they allow you to stay distracted from eating by making you feel fuller. By ingesting protein, the primary energy source is shifted from carbohydrate to fat. It is similar to ketosis (adapted to fat consumption), where you can use your body fat instead of carbohydrate.

How to Start the Diet?

Although it is as simple as a diet can be, the initial weeks can be hard. Here are the things that you can incorporate to get through the changeover conveniently:

- Before starting with the diet, you can get your blood test done since the metabolic needs vary with every individual.

- You might feel like giving up at some point, start getting headaches, and experience fatigue. It is normal as your body will be getting used to using energy from fat rather than carbohydrates.

- Your eating desire might fluctuate. You will get adjusted to this form of eating after one week.

Chapter 2: Recipes for Tasty Appetizers

If you are a meat lover and want to start the carnivore diet, here are some recipes for you to follow.

Oven-Baked Chicken Wings

Total Prep & Cooking Time: 1 hour 5 minutes

Yields: 8 servings

Nutrition Facts: Calories: 348 | Carbs: 1g | Protein: 25g | Fat: 27g | Fiber: 1g

Ingredients:

- Half cup of grated Parmesan
- Four pounds of chicken wings
- One tsp. of salt
- One tbsp. of parsley
- A quarter cup of grass-fed butter
- Half tsp. of black pepper (ground)

Method:

1. First of all, the oven needs to be preheated to 180 degrees Celsius or 350 degrees Fahrenheit.

2. Take a parchment paper for lining the baking sheet.

3. Now, you need to take a shallow bowl or dish for melting the butter.

4. In another clean bowl, mix parsley, pepper, Parmesan cheese, and salt.

5. Once the herb and cheese mixture is ready, dip the chicken wings in the bowl of melted butter one by one. After dipping, roll the wings in the mixture.

6. Arrange all the wings properly on top of the baking sheet.

7. Bake for an hour.

8. Take out the baked chicken wings from the oven and serve them warm.

Steak Nuggets

Total Prep & Cooking Time: 55-60 minutes

Yields: 4 servings

Nutrition Facts: Calories: 350 | Carbs: 1g | Protein: 40g | Fat: 20g | Fiber: 2g

Ingredients:

- One pound of beefsteak or venison steak (cut it into chunks)
- Palm or lard oil (needed for frying)
- One large-sized egg

For Keto Breading,

- Half cup each of
  - Pork panko
  - Parmesan cheese (grated)
- Half tsp. of seasoned salt (homemade)

For Chipotle Ranch Dip,

- A quarter cup each of
  - Organic cultured cream (sour)
  - Mayonnaise
- More than one tsp. of chipotle paste (for taste)
- A quarter medium-sized lime (juiced)

Method:

1. For preparing the Chipotle Ranch Dip, you need to combine all the ingredients and mix properly. Use either more or less chipotle paste in accordance to your taste preference. Refrigerate the dip before serving for a minimum of thirty minutes. You may store the dip for nearly a week.

2. Take a large-sized bowl and combine parmesan cheese, seasoned salt, and pork panko. Set aside after mixing evenly.

3. Now, beat one egg. Place the breading mix in one bowl and beaten egg in another.

4. Dip the steak chunks first in egg and then in the breading mix. Then, place them on a plate or sheet pan lined with wax paper.

5. Before frying, freeze the raw breaded steak bites for half an hour. By doing so, the breading won't lift at the time of frying.

6. Heat the lard to 325 degrees Fahrenheit. Fry the chilled or frozen steak nuggets for nearly two to three minutes until you get the brown color.

7. Keep the fried nuggets on a plate lined with a paper towel. Sprinkle a pinch of salt. Serve hot along with Chipotle Ranch.

Grilled Shrimp

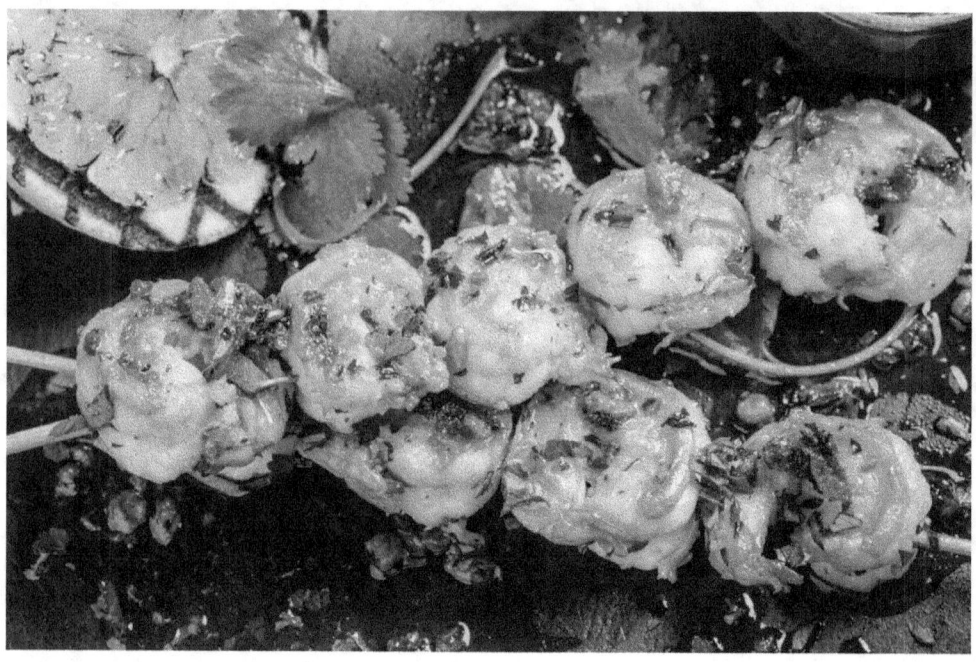

Total Prep & Cooking Time: 10 minutes

Yields: 4 servings

Nutrition Facts: Calories: 102 | Carbs: 1g | Protein: 28g | Fat: 3g | Fiber: 0g

Ingredients:

For grilling,

- One lb. of shrimp
- One tbsp. of lemon juice (freshly squeezed)

- Two tbsps. of olive oil (extra-virgin)
- For frying – vegetable oil or canola oil

For the shrimp seasoning,

- Half a tsp. of cayenne pepper
- One tsp. each of
  - Italian seasoning
  - Kosher salt
  - Garlic powder

Method:

1. You have to preheat your grill for this recipe on high.

2. Take a mixing bowl of large size, add all the ingredients of the seasoning in it and mix them well. Drizzle the lemon juice and olive oil into the mixture and keep stirring until you get a paste.

3. Add the shrimp into the bowl of seasonings and keep tossing so that all the pieces are evenly coated. Take the shrimp pieces and thread them onto wooden skewers.

4. Coat your grill with canola oil. You have to grill the shrimp for about three minutes for each side until they become opaque and pink.

5. Serve and enjoy!

Notes: *You can store the grilled shrimp in the refrigerator for up to three days if you want to, but for the best flavor, you should consume it on the same day.*

Roasted Bone Marrow

Total Prep & Cooking Time: 20 minutes

Yields: 2 servings

Nutrition Facts: Calories: 440 | Carbs: 0g | Protein: 4g | Fat: 48g | Fiber: 0g

Ingredients:

- To season – freshly ground black pepper and sea salt flakes
- Four bone marrow halves

Method:

1. Set the temperature of your oven to 350 degrees F and preheat.
2. Take a baking tray with deep sides and then place the bone marrow pieces in it.
3. Bake the bone marrow for half an hour until they become crispy and golden brown in color. The fat that is present in excess should have rendered off by now.
4. Season with black pepper and sea salt flakes.
5. You can spread the marrow separately on top of steaks, or you can serve the bone marrow as an appetizer.

Bacon-Wrapped Chicken Bites

Total Prep & Cooking Time: 30 minutes

Yields: 4 servings

Nutrition Facts: Calories: 230 | Carbs: 5g | Protein: 22g | Fat: 13g | Fiber: 1g

Ingredients:

- Three tbsps. of garlic powder
- Eight slices of thin bacon (slice them into one-third pieces)
- One chicken breast (large-sized, cut into bite-sized pieces)

Method:

1. Set the temperature of the oven to 400 degrees F and use aluminum foil to line the baking tray—Preheat the oven.
2. In a bowl, add the garlic powder. Take each chicken piece and dip it into the garlic powder.
3. Now, take each short piece of bacon and wrap it around the piece of chicken. Keep these prepared chicken pieces on the baking tray. Make sure they are not touching each other.
4. Bake the preparation for half an hour, and by the end of it, the bacon should turn crispy. After about fifteen minutes through pieces, turn the pieces over.

Salami Egg Muffins

Total Prep & Cooking Time: 25 minutes

Yields: 12 servings

Nutrition Facts: Calories: 142 | Carbs: 1g | Protein: 12g | Fat: 10g | Fiber: 0g

Ingredients:

- Four eggs (large-sized)
- Twenty slices of salami (uncured)
- Half a tsp. of kosher salt
- A quarter tsp. of black pepper
- Olive oil

Method:

1. Set the temperature of the oven to 350 degrees F and preheat. Take ramekins of four ounces each and spray them with olive oil. Then, place these ramekins on the baking sheet.

2. On the bottom of each ramekin, place one slice of salami and then on the sides, arrange four slices so that they are overlapping each other.

3. In this way, you will get a basket of salami, and in the middle of the basket, break one egg. Form four such baskets. Season the baskets with pepper and salt.

4. Bake the prepared salami baskets for twenty minutes, and by that time, they should be set.

5. Around the edges of the muffins, run a knife, and the muffins will get released. Serve and enjoy!

3-Ingredients Scotch Eggs

Total Prep & Cooking Time: 40 minutes

Yields: 12 servings

Nutrition Facts: Calories: 270 | Carbs: 1g | Protein: 19g | Fat: 20g | Fiber: 5g

Ingredients:

- Twelve large-sized boiled eggs
- Two pounds of chicken sausage or ground beef
- Two tsps. of salt

Method:

1. Preheating the oven to a temperature of 175 degrees Celsius or 350 degrees Fahrenheit is the first step for preparing such a delicious appetizer.

2. Line two baking sheets (small rimmed) with a parchment paper.

3. Take a large-sized bowl and combine chicken or beef and salt. Mix both the ingredients together by using your hands and then form twelve meatballs with it. Press the meatballs flat after placing them on top of the lined sheets.

4. Now, place each boiled egg inside each circle of flattened meat. After placing the eggs, start wrapping the meat nicely around the eggs. You are not supposed to leave any holes or gaps.

5. You need to bake for nearly fifteen minutes. Flip over as soon as the top looks cooked and again bake for ten minutes. If you want a crispy shell, then finish it under a broiler for approximately five minutes.

Notes: *If you are willing to enhance the taste, then you may feel free to add any of your favorite herbs, such as garlic or rosemary powder. Add one tsp. of your preferred herb into the meat just before wrapping the eggs. Hard-boiled eggs are better in this case as it is difficult to peel the soft boiled eggs.*

Chapter 3: Quick and Easy Everyday Recipes

Carnivore Waffles
Total Prep & Cooking Time: 6 minutes

Yields: 1 serving

Nutrition Facts: Calories: 274 | Carbs: 1g | Protein: 23.6g | Fat: 20.2g | Fiber: 0.8g

Ingredients:

- One-third cup of mozzarella cheese
- One egg
- Half cup of pork rinds (ground)
- A pinch of salt

Method:

1. For preparing the carnivore waffles, all you need is a waffle maker. First of all, preheat your waffle maker (medium-high heat).

2. Take a medium-sized bowl and whisk the pork rinds, cheese, and salt together.

3. Once you are done with the whisking part, pour the already prepared waffle mixture in the middle of the waffle maker's iron.

4. Close it and allow it to cook for three to five minutes. Or, you may cook until the waffle gets an attractive golden brown color.

5. Now, remove the cooked waffle and serve hot.

Notes: *The carnivore waffle will turn out to be more delicious if you place a cube of butter or runny egg on top of it. Greasing the waffle maker is not required before you start cooking waffles.*

Chicken Bacon Pancakes

Total Prep & Cooking Time: 20 minutes

Yields: 4 servings

Nutrition Facts: Calories: 444 | Carbs: 0g | Protein: 33g | Fat: 34g | Fiber: 0g

Ingredients:

- Four bacon slices
- Two chicken breasts
- Two tbsps. of coconut oil
- Four eggs (medium-sized, whisked)

Method:

1. First, you need to add all the ingredients to the bowl of the food processor except for the oil and then process everything together to form a smooth mixture.
2. After that, take your frying pan, and coconut oil to it.
3. From the batter that you just made, form four pancakes.
4. Fry these pancakes until they are set and properly cooked. Do the same with the rest of the batter.

Garlic Cilantro Salmon

Total Prep & Cooking Time: 25 minutes

Yields: 4 servings

Nutrition Facts: Calories: 294 | Carbs: 1g | Protein: 38.9g | Fat: 14.2g | Fiber: 0g

Ingredients:

- One lemon
- One fillet of salmon (large)
- A quarter cup of cilantro leaves (freshly chopped)
- Four garlic cloves (minced)
- One tablespoon of butter (optional)
- To taste – freshly ground black pepper and kosher salt

Method:

1. Set the temperature of the oven to 400 degrees F and preheat. Take a baking sheet and line it with foil. Place the fillets of salmon on it. You don't have to grease the foil.

2. Sprinkle the juice of one lemon over the fillet of salmon. Spread cilantro and garlic on top of the fillets evenly and season with pepper and salt. If

you want to use butter, then you have to place thin slices on top of the salmon fillet at this stage.

3. Now, place the salmon along with the foil in the oven and bake for about seven minutes.

4. Set broil settings and cook the salmon for an additional seven minutes. The top part should become crispy.

5. Use a flat spatula to remove the salmon from the oven. Separate the skin from the fish and serve!

Mustard-Seared Bacon Burgers

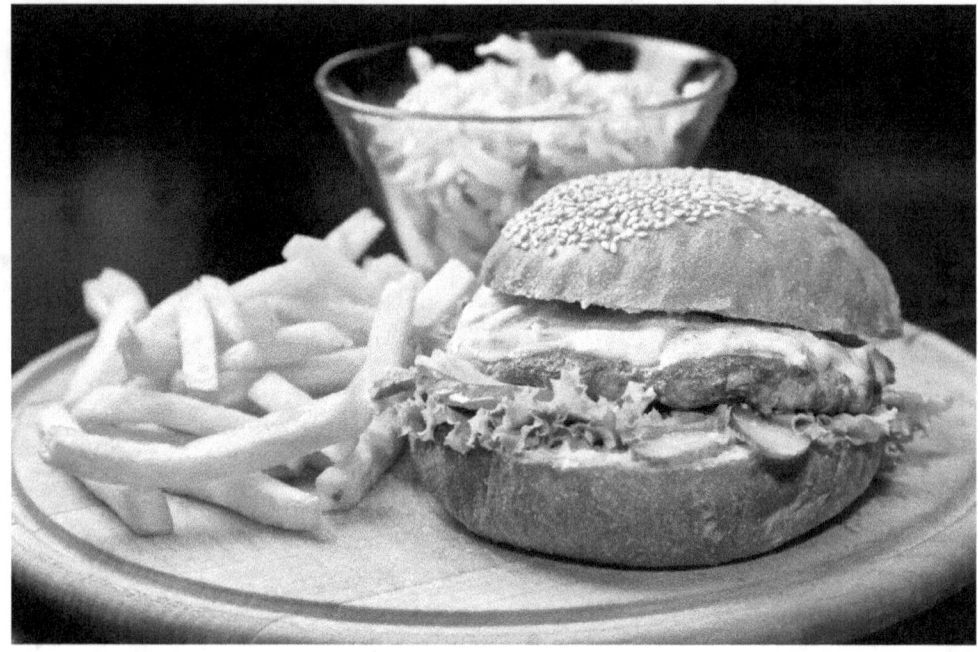

Total Prep & Cooking Time: 30 minutes

Yields: 6 servings

Nutrition Facts: Calories: 525 | Carbs: 3g | Protein: 22g | Fat: 45g | Fiber: 4g

Ingredients:

- 1.5 pounds of ground beef
- Four ounces of diced bacon
- Six tbsps. of yellow mustard
- To taste – salt and pepper

For the toppings,

- One tomato (properly diced)
- Half a red onion (diced)
- One avocado (thinly sliced)

For the sauce,

- Two tsps. of yellow mustard
- One tsp. of tomato paste
- A quarter cup of mayo

Method:

1. Take a pan and cook the bacon in it until it becomes crispy. You have to keep the grease of the bacon separately so that it can be used later. Then, take the bacon bits and keep them in a bowl along with the ground beef. Use pepper and salt to season them.

2. You will be able to form six patties from the mixture.

3. Now, you have to fry these burger patties on high flame so that they can get a great color. If you want, you can also choose to grill them.

4. Each patty will then have to be coated with one tbsp. of mustard and then, place the patty on the pan with the mustard-side facing down. Sear the patties one by one.

5. Take another bowl in which you can mix all the ingredients of the sauce together.

6. Each burger patty will have to be coated with sauce, and then, you can top them with slices of avocado, tomato, and onions.

Crockpot Shredded Chicken

Total Prep & Cooking Time: 6 hours

Yields: 8 servings

Nutrition Facts: Calories: 201 | Carbs: 1g | Protein: 24g | Fat: 10g | Fiber: 0g

Ingredients:

- Four garlic cloves
- Four chicken breasts
- One cup of chicken broth
- Half an onion (sliced)
- One tbsp. of Italian seasoning
- To taste – Salt and pepper

Method:

1. Take all the ingredients and add them to the crockpot.
2. Cook them for about six hours on low.
3. Use forks to shred the meat.
4. You can enjoy the shredded chicken with a variety of dishes like sautés, lettuce wraps, salads, or even soups.

Chapter 4: Weekend Dinner Recipes

Organ Meat Pie

Total Prep & Cooking Time: 20 minutes

Yields: 4 servings

Nutrition Facts: Calories: 412 | Carbs: 2g | Protein: 35g | Fat: 28g | Fiber: 4.2g

Ingredients:

- Half pound each of
  - Beef liver (ground)
  - Beef heart (ground)
  - Ground beef
- Three eggs
- Butter, ghee or Homemade Tallow or any melted cooking fat
- Salt (as required)

Method:

1. The oven needs to be preheated to 175 degrees Celsius or 350 degrees Fahrenheit.

2. Take a mixing bowl: mix ground beef, beef heart, and beef liver along with eggs and cooking fat of your choice. Lastly, add salt into the mixture.

3. Now, take a pie plate of nine inches and grease it lightly. Pour the mixture into the pie plate evenly.

4. Bake it for nearly fifteen to twenty minutes. Or, you may bake until the egg is totally set.

5. After baking, remove the pie from direct heat and let it cool for about five minutes. Serve it in a warm condition. In the case of leftovers, enjoy it cold.

Notes: *For those of you who are willing to add flavor to this recipe, you may add half tbsp. of any seasoning mix with the meat.*

Smokey Bacon Meatballs

Total Prep & Cooking Time: 30 minutes

Yields: 8 servings

Nutrition Facts: Calories: 280 | Carbs: 1g | Protein: 13g | Fat: 25g | Fiber: 0g

Ingredients:

- Two garlic cloves (skins peeled)
- Eight bacon slices (crumbled and cooked)
- One pound ground chicken or two chicken breasts
- One egg (properly whisked)
- Two drops of liquid smoke
- One tbsp. of onion powder
- Four tbsps. of olive oil

Method:

1. First, take all the ingredients (except for the oil) and add them to the bowl of the food processor and mix everything.

2. You will be able to form about twenty to twenty-four meatballs from the mixture. These balls will be small in size.

3. Now, take a large-sized frying pan, and then heat the oil. Add the meatballs and fry them until they are browned. It will take about five minutes for each side. If you want them to be perfect, then avoid overcrowding and cook in batches.

Steak au Poivre

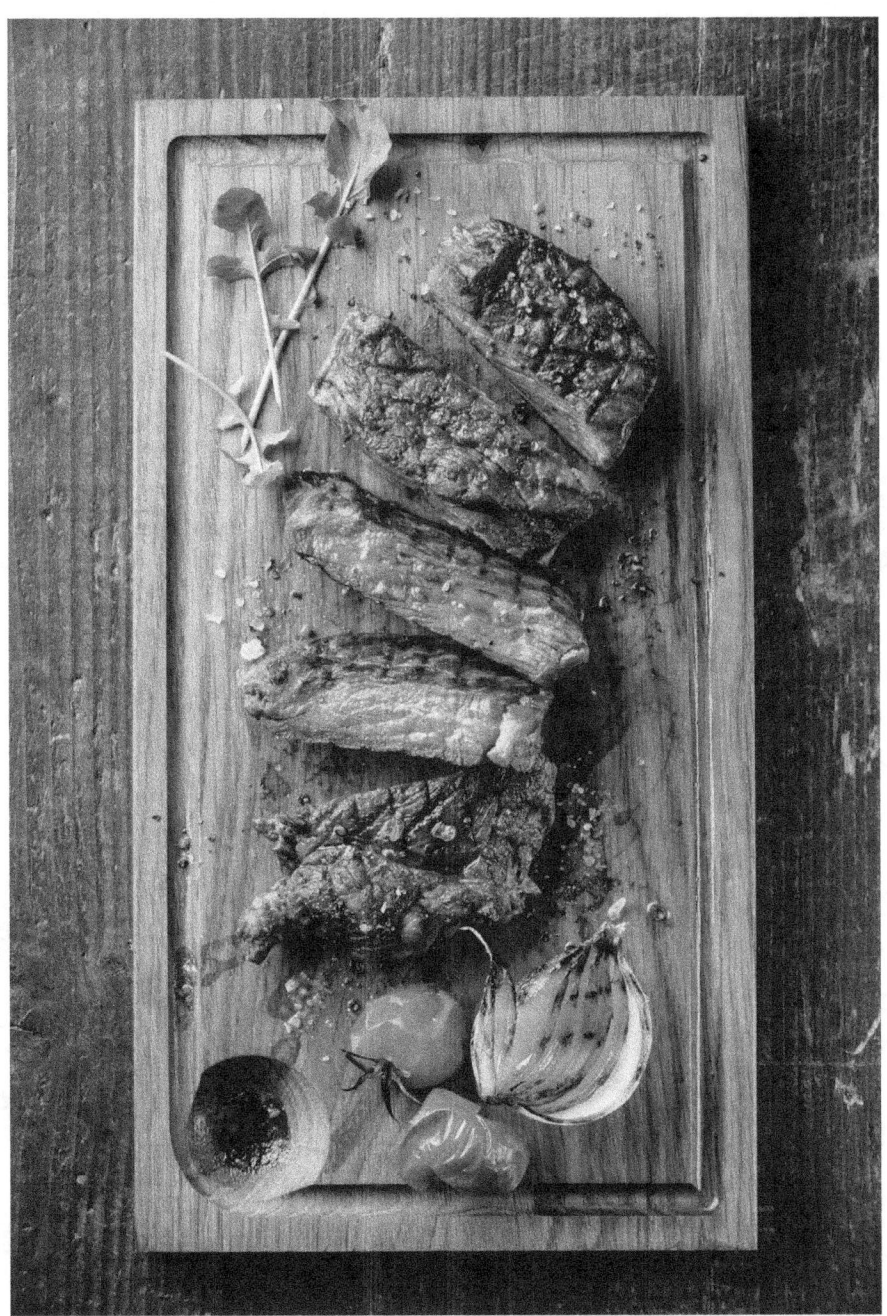

Total Prep & Cooking Time: 15 minutes

Yields: 1 serving

Nutrition Facts: Calories: 696 | Carbs: 2g | Protein: 42g | Fat: 58g | Fiber: 0g

Ingredients:

- One fillet of mignon (approximately six ounces)
- One thyme sprig
- One tbsp. of salt
- Two tbsps. each of
    - Ghee
    - Peppercorns
- Two garlic cloves (minced)

Method:

1. After you take the steaks out of the refrigerator, season them nicely with salt and then allow them to sit for about half an hour.

2. Use a mortar and pestle to crush the peppercorns completely on a pan or a flat board.

3. Take the steak, and on both sides of it, press the crushed peppercorns.

4. Place a skillet on the oven and heat it. Add the ghee. After that, sauté the thyme and garlic.

5. When you notice that the ghee has become hot, place the pieces of steak in the pan. Cook each side for about four minutes. The end result will be medium-rare steak.

Skillet Rib Eye Steaks

Total Prep & Cooking Time: 55 minutes

Yields: 2 servings

Nutrition Facts: Calories: 347 | Carbs: 1g | Protein: 22g | Fat: 14.2g | Fiber: 0g

Ingredients:

- Two tsps. of freshly chopped rosemary leaves
- One tsp. of seasoning of your choice
- One tbsp. each of
  - Olive oil
  - Unsalted butter
- One rib-eye steak (bone-in)

Method:

1. Take the sheet pan and on it, place the rib-eye steak. Use the seasoning to coat both sides properly. Spread the rosemary leaves on top.

2. Now, keep this steak in the refrigerator for three days after covering. Before cooking, take the steak out and keep it outside at room temperature for half an hour.

3. Place a skillet on the oven and heat it. Add olive oil and butter and wait until all of the butter has melted. Coat the skillet properly with butter by tilting the pan.

4. Now, add the steak to the skillet and cook for about five minutes until you notice that the bottom side has become caramelized and browned. After that, flip it over and baste the other side with oil and butter and cook it for five more minutes.

5. Take the steak off from the pan and slice it into thin pieces after it has cooled down for about five minutes.

Pan-Fried Pork Tenderloin

Total Prep & Cooking Time: 20 minutes

Yields: 2 servings

Nutrition Facts: Calories: 330 | Carbs: 0g | Protein: 47g | Fat: 15g | Fiber: 0g

Ingredients:

- One tbsp. of coconut oil
- To taste – pepper and salt
- One pound of pork tenderloin

Method:

1. Start by cutting the pork tenderloin in two halves.
2. Place your frying pan on the oven on medium flame. Add the oil in the pan and heat it.
3. Once the oil has melted completely, place the two pieces of the pork tenderloin in the oil.
4. Allow the pieces to cook thoroughly. Use tongs to flip the pieces so that all the sides of the pork are evenly cooked.
5. Take a reading on the thermometer, and it should show that the temperature is just below 63 degrees C or 145 degrees F.
6. Allow the pork to cool down after you take it out and then use a sharp knife to cut it into small pieces.

Carnivore Chicken Enchiladas

Total Prep & Cooking Time: 30 minutes

Yields: 10 servings

Nutrition Facts: Calories: 271 | Carbs: 5g | Protein: 25g | Fat: 7g | Fiber: 1.5g

Ingredients:

- Two chicken breasts (skinless, boneless)
- Three tbsps. of bottles lime juice + juice of one fresh lime
- One tsp. of dried garlic
- 16 oz. of sliced chicken
- Chimichurri sauce
- One jar of enchilada sauce
- One bell pepper (thinly sliced)
- Eight oz. each of
    - Cooked spinach
    - Shredded cheese

Method:

For making the shredded chicken,

1. First, take a crockpot and add the shredded pieces of chicken in it. Add the lime juice too.

2. Sprinkle the Chimichurri sauce on top of the chicken and then sprinkle the garlic on top.

3. Now, cook the chicken for about 4-5 hours if you want to cook it on high. Alternatively, if you're going to cook it on low, then set it for 8 hours.

4. Once it is done, use a fork to shred the chicken.

Assembling the enchiladas,

1. Set the temperature of your oven to 400 degrees F and preheat.

2. Take all the other ingredients like pepper and spinach and prep them.

3. The enchilada wrapped will be made by the four slices of chicken.

4. In the middle of the wrapper, add the shredded chicken.

5. Then, on either side, add the cooked spinach, pepper, and some of the cheese.

6. Roll the wrappers carefully and make sure they are firm.

7. Once you have rolled them completely, place them in a pan with the seam sides facing downwards. Then, add the enchilada sauce all over them.

8. Take the remaining portion of the cheese and sprinkle on top of the enchiladas. Bake the preparation for about fifteen minutes in the oven.

9. Serve and enjoy!

PART III

You will find many of the Chinese recipes will call for shoyu. Shoyu is the term broadly given to soy sauces that are made from fermented soybeans, wheat, salt, and water. In general, they are quite thin and clear and are excellent as an all-purpose cooking and table sauce. One of the best selling shoyu in the world is proclaimed to be Kikkoman Soy Sauce.

Chapter 1: Soup

Hot & Sour Soup

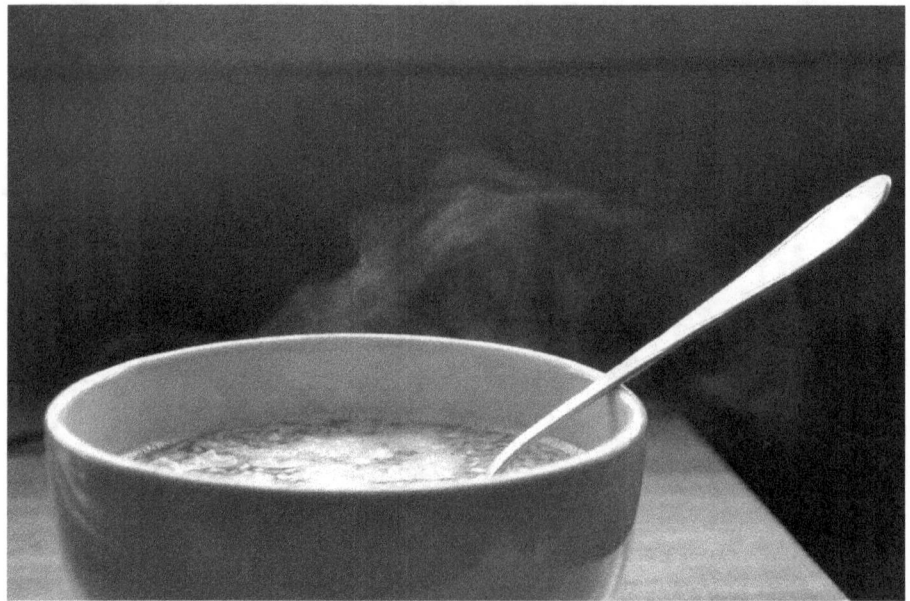

Servings Provided: 4

Time Required: 40 minutes

What is Needed:

- Chicken broth - low-sodium (1 quart)
- Dried tree ear fungus (.25 cup)
- Dried lily buds (12)

- Medium-dark soy sauce (2 tbsp. + more for seasoning)
- Distilled white vinegar (2 tbsp. + more for seasoning)
- Cornstarch (2 tbsp.)
- Kosher salt (.5 tsp.)
- Large eggs (2)
- Bamboo shoots (.5 cup - shredded)
- Cooked pork, ham, or chicken (.5 cup - shredded)
- Spiced thick - dry tofu - shredded (1 cup/3.5 oz.)
- White pepper - finely ground (1.5 tsp.)
- Sesame oil (1 tbsp.)
- To serve: Chopped cilantro & scallions

Preparation Method:

1. Dump the lily buds into boiling water to soak about ten minutes until they're softened. Discard the rough tips.
2. Prepare another container and add the tree fungus and boiling water to soak from 20 minutes to half an hour. Rinse, drain, and coarsely chop them.
3. Dump the broth into a large saucepan. Once boiling, add the soy sauce, salt, and vinegar.
4. Whisk three tablespoons of water with the cornstarch and mix it into the broth to simmer for three to four minutes to thicken.
5. Once it's at a rolling boil, whisk the eggs and a dash of salt, and work it into the soup in a circular fashion. Wait five seconds, stir and extinguish the heat.
6. Toss in the tofu, chicken, white pepper, bamboo shoots, ear fungus, and lily buds.
7. Simmer the soup using the medium temperature setting for about two minutes, adding in vinegar, soy sauce, and salt as desired.
8. Portion the soup and garnish it using the cilantro, scallions, and a spritz of sesame oil.

Wonton Soup

Servings Provided: 8

Time Required: 1 hour 15 minutes

What is Needed:

- Pork - fresh loin - whole (.5 lb.)
- Crustaceans - shrimp - mixed-species - raw (2 oz.)
- Brown sugar (1 tsp.)
- Burgundy wine (1 tbsp.)
- Shoyu - low-sodium soy sauce (1 tbsp.)
- Spring onions/scallions - tops & bulb (1 tsp.)
- Ginger root (1 tsp.)
- Wonton wrappers - includes egg roll wrappers (24 @ 3.5-inch square)
- Clear chicken broth - Swanson - CAM (3 cups)
- Scallions (includes tops and bulb- (1/8 cup)

Preparation Method:

1. Chop the green onion and add one teaspoon into a large mixing container and add the pork, shrimp, sugar, wine, shoyu sauce, and ginger. Thoroughly toss the mixture and let stand for 25 to 30 minutes.
2. Scoop the filling (1 tsp.) into the middle of each wonton skin.
3. Moisten the four edges of the wonton wrapper with a small amount of water on your fingertips, and pull the top corner down to the bottom, folding the wrapper over the filling to create a triangle.
4. Seal it by pressing the edges firmly. Bring the left and right corners together above the filling and overlap the corner of the tips. Moisten with water and press together. Repeat the process until all wrappers are used.
5. Make the soup. Heat the chicken stock to a rolling boil. Add the wontons and cook for five minutes.
6. Top off the soup with chopped green onions and serve.

Chapter 2: Seafood

Honey Walnut Shrimp

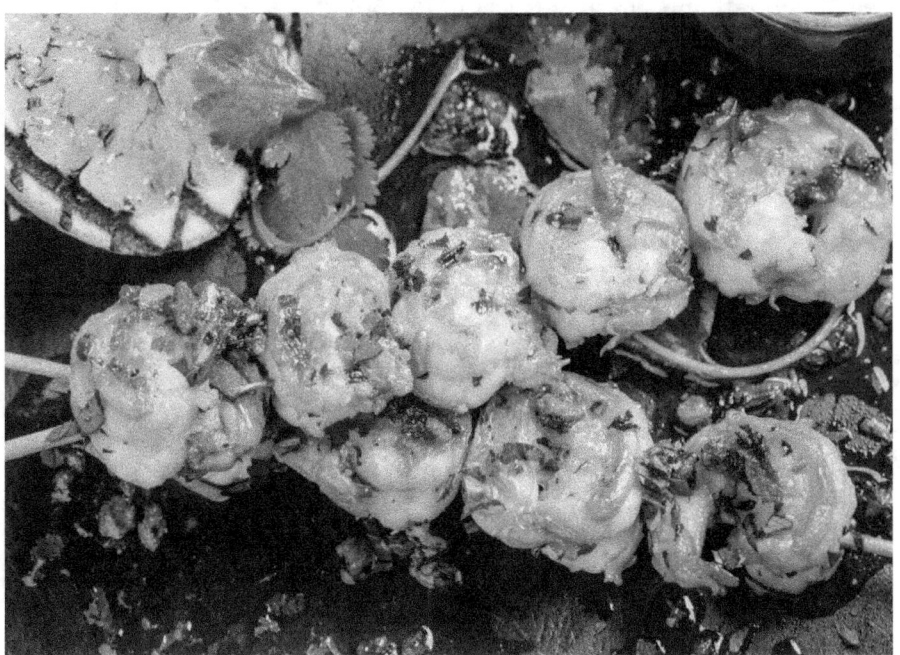

Servings Provided: 4

Time Required: 30 minutes

What is Needed:

- Water (1 cup)
- English walnuts (.5 cup)
- Granulated sugar (2/3 cup)

- Egg white - raw (4)
- Rice flour - white (2/3 cup)
- Salad dressing/soybean oil with salt/mayonnaise (.25 cup)
- Jumbo shrimp - fresh & raw (1 lb./21-30)
- Honey - strained or extracted (2 tbsp.)
- Sweet condensed canned milk (1 tbsp.)
- Oil for frying (1 cup)

Preparation Method:

1. Whisk the water and sugar in a small saucepan. Once boiling, add the walnuts and boil them for two minutes. Dump them into a colander to drain. Arrange the nuts on a baking tray to thoroughly dry.
2. Whip the egg whites in a mixing container until they're foamy. Stir in the mochiko until it's a pasty consistency.
3. Warm the oil using the med-high temperature setting in a heavy deep skillet.
4. Dip the shrimp into the batter, and fry them until nicely browned (5 min.). Transfer them to a paper towel-lined platter using a slotted spoon to allow them to drain.
5. Whisk the honey, mayonnaise, and sweetened condensed milk. Fold in the shrimp and toss to coat with the sauce.
6. Garnish using the candied walnuts right before serving.

Steamed Fish

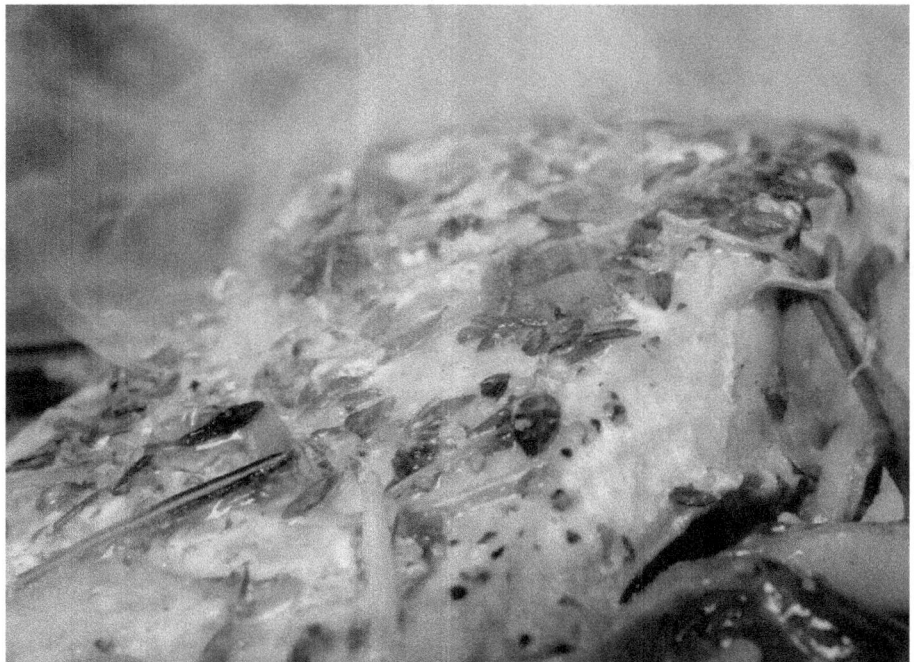

Servings Provided: 2

Time Required: 35 minutes

What is Needed:

- Raw finfish, snapper, mixed species (1 lb.)
- Salt (.5 tsp.)
- Black pepper (.5 tsp.)
- Ginger root - raw (1 tbsp.)
- Shoyu soy sauce (1 tbsp.)
- Sesame oil (2 tsp.)
- Shiitake mushrooms - raw AMM (2)

- Tomatoes (1 fresh)
- Peppers - raw red-hot chile (half of 1)
- Cilantro (2 sprigs - raw)

Preparation Method:

1. Prepare a steamer with a basket large enough for the snapper to lie flat. Pour in 1.5 inches of water and wait for it to boil.
2. Sprinkle the snapper with pepper and salt and pepper before placing it into the basket. Top the fish with ginger, and drizzle with sesame oil and soy sauce.
3. Place the tomatoes, mushrooms, and red chile pepper in the steamer basket.
4. Set a timer and steam the fish for 15 minutes, or until easily flaked with a fork. Garnish with cilantro and serve.

Stir-Fried Shrimp & Scallions

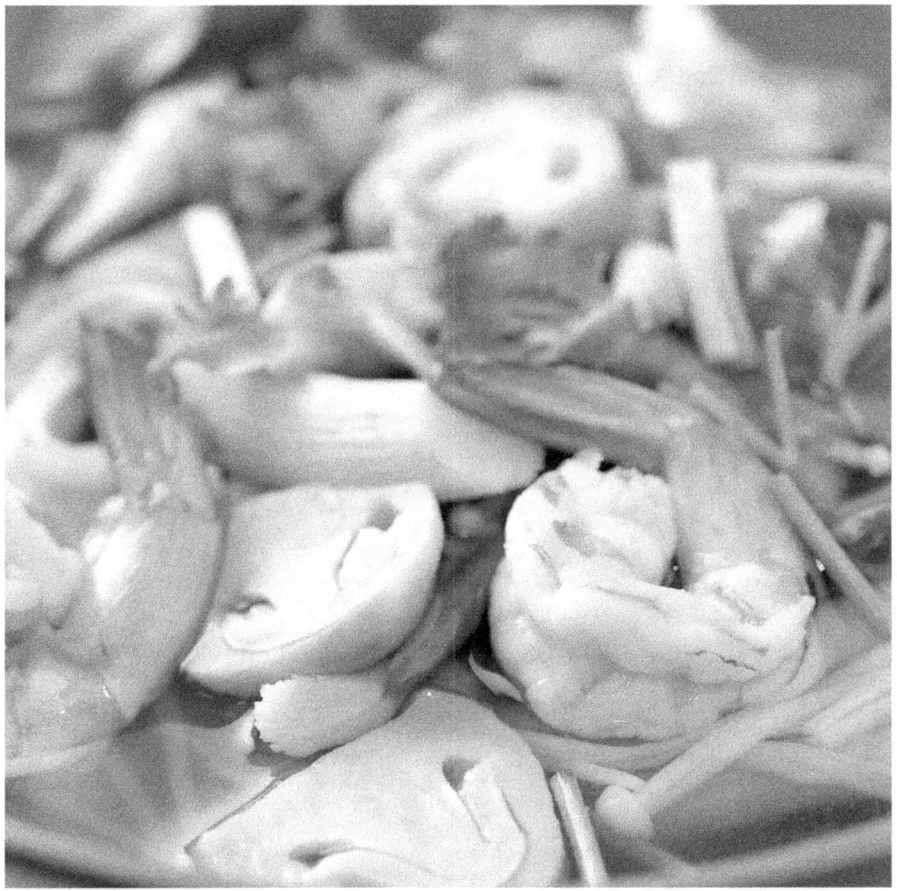

Servings Provided: 4

Time Required: 30 minutes

What is Needed:

- Jumbo shrimp (1.5 lb.)

- Garlic (3 cloves)
- Fresh ginger (1-inch section)
- Crushed red pepper (1.5 tsp.)
- Egg white (1 large)
- Cornstarch (2 tsp. - divided)
- Ketchup (.75 cup)
- Chicken broth - low-sodium (.5 cup)
- Black pepper & kosher salt (1.5 tsp. each)
- Sugar (1 tbsp.)
- Canola oil (.25 cup)
- Chopped cilantro (.5 cup)
- Scallions (3)

Preparation Method:

1. Thinly slice the scallions. Shell and devein the shrimp. Mince the garlic and ginger.
2. Toss the shrimp with the ginger, garlic, red pepper, one teaspoon of the cornstarch, and egg white until well-coated.
3. Whisk the broth with the ketchup, sugar, salt, and pepper with the rest of the cornstarch.
4. Warm a large skillet with the oil until it shimmers. Add the shrimp and stir-fry using the high-temperature setting until pink.
5. Add the ketchup mixture and simmer until the shrimp are heated (2 min.). Stir in the cilantro and scallions to serve.

Chapter 3: Poultry

Kung Pao Chicken - Keto-Friendly

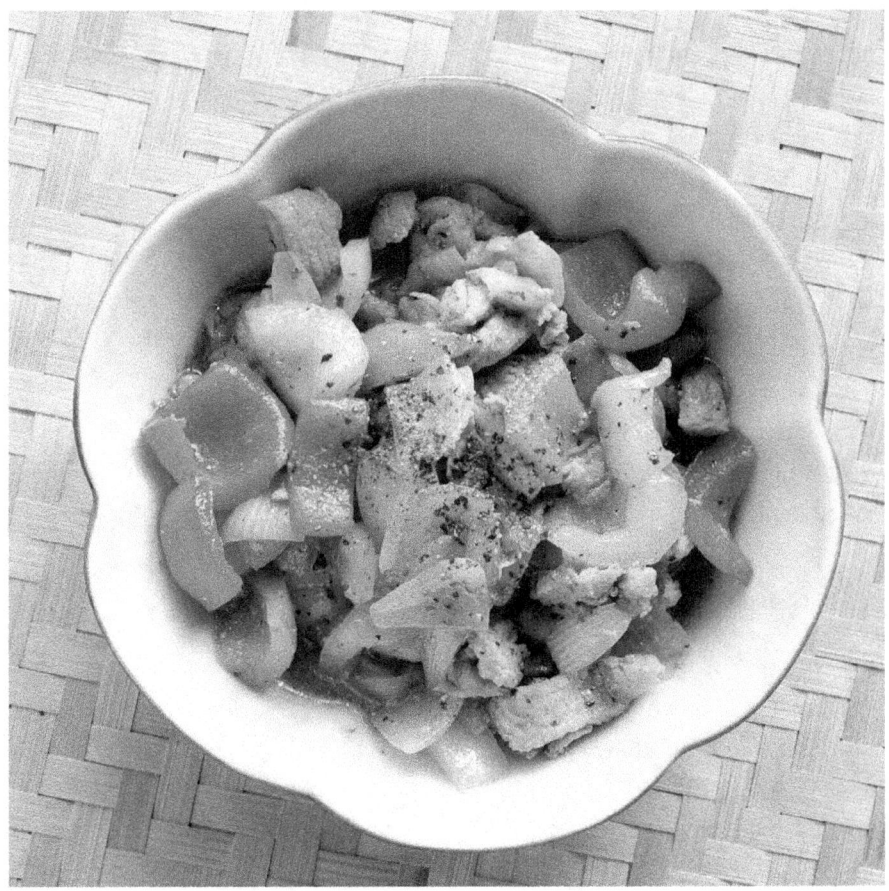

Servings Provided: 4

Time Required: 40 minutes

What is Needed:

- Chicken breasts - boneless skinless (1 lb.)
  The Marinade:

- Chinese rice wine/dry sherry (2 tsp.)
- Soy sauce (2 tsp.)
- Cornstarch (2 tsp.)

To Cook:

- Olive oil or sunflower oil (3 tbsp. divided)
- Dried red chilies (4-6)
- Green onions (4)
- Optional: Red finger chili (1)
- Asparagus (1 bunch)
- Sweet bell pepper (1)
- Garlic & ginger (4 tsp. each)
- Mini cucumbers (2)
- Roasted salted peanuts/cashews (.33 cup)
- Toasted sesame seeds (1 tsp.)

The Sauce:

- Water (3 tbsp. - cold)
- Soy sauce & white vinegar (2 tbsp. each)
- Chinese wine/ sherry (1 tbsp.)
- Cornstarch (2 tsp.)
- Salt (.5 tsp.)
- Optional: Asian chili-garlic sauce (1 tbsp.)

Preparation Method:

1. Slice the chicken into one-inch chunks and combine it with the marinade fixings in the first group (soy sauce, rice wine, and cornstarch) stirring to combine. Marinate the mixture for 15 minutes.
2. Prep the veggies by cutting the asparagus into large pieces and mincing the garlic and onion. Chop the cucumber. Core and cube the bell pepper. Cut the green onions into one-inch pieces.

3. Prepare a large-sized cast-iron pan to warm one tablespoon of oil using the med-high temperature setting. Add the green onions, dried chilies, and finger chili.
4. Simmer the mixture until the green onions are slightly charred (1 min.). Transfer them to a baking sheet or large platter.
5. Heat the rest of the oil in the pan (1 tbsp.). Add asparagus and bell pepper and cook, stirring until it's slightly charred (2-3 min.).
6. Transfer to a baking tray and add the remainder of the oil (1.5 tsp.) to the pan. Working in two batches, stir-fry the chicken until browned (3-4 min. per batch), repeating with remaining oil.
7. Make the Sauce: Whisk the water, rice wine, soy sauce, and cornstarch until smooth. Return the chicken, vegetables, and chilies to the pan.
8. Sprinkle with salt, stir in the sauce, and cook until the liquid is bubbling and thickened (30 seconds to one minute). Stir in the cucumbers, peanuts, and chili-garlic sauce.
9. Serve it with a garnish of sesame seeds.

Orange Chicken

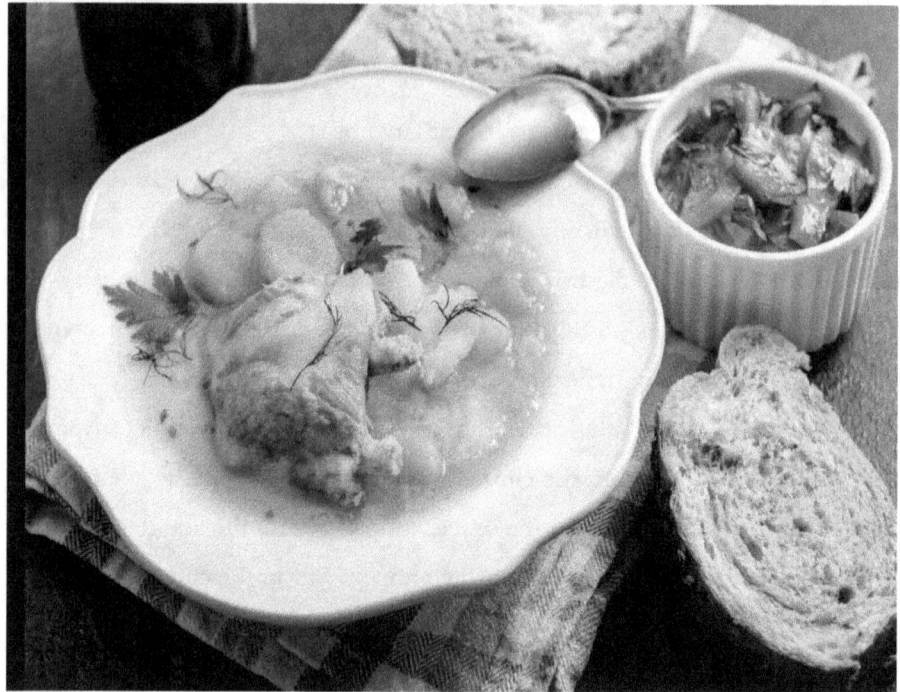

Servings Provided: 4

Time Required: 35 minutes

What is Needed:

The Chicken:

- Oil (as needed for frying)
- Boneless & skinless chicken breasts (4)
- Eggs (3 whisked)
- Cornstarch (.33 cup)
- Flour (.33 cup)
  Orange Chicken Sauce:

- Orange juice (1 cup)
- Sugar (.5 cup)
- Rice/white vinegar (2 tbsp.)

- Tamari or soy sauce (2 tbsp.)
- Ginger (.25 tsp.)
- Garlic powder (.25 tsp.) or 2 garlic cloves (2 finely diced)
- Red chili flakes (.5 tsp.)
- Orange Zest (1 orange)
- Cornstarch (1 tbsp.)
  The Garnish:

- Orange Zest
- Green Onions

Preparation Method:

1. Prepare the orange sauce. Mince the ginger and garlic. Pour the vinegar, orange juice, soy sauce, sugar, garlic, ginger, and red chili flakes into a saucepan. Sauté them for about three minutes.
2. Whisk one tablespoon of cornstarch with two tablespoons of water to form a paste. Add it to the orange sauce and whisk thoroughly. Continue cooking the sauce for about five minutes, until the mixture begins to thicken. After it's thickened, remove the pan from the burner and add the orange zest.
3. Prepare the chicken by cutting it into bite-sized chunks.
4. Dump the flour, a pinch of salt, and cornstarch in a pie plate or another shallow dish.
5. Whisk eggs in a shallow mixing container.
6. Dip the pieces of chicken into the egg mix and then flour mixture. Place them onto a platter.
7. Next, warm two to three inches of oil in a heavy-bottomed skillet (med-high temperature). Use an electric skillet or use a thermometer to check the heat until it reaches 350° Fahrenheit.
8. Working in batches, fry several chicken pieces at a time. Cook them for two to three minutes, often turning until golden brown, and place the chicken on a paper-towel-lined plate. Repeat the process until all the chicken is cooked.
9. Toss the chicken with the orange sauce. Reserve some of the sauce to serve over the rice. Serve it with a sprinkling of green onion and orange zest to your liking.

Chapter 4: Pork

Chinese Pork BBQ (Char Siu)

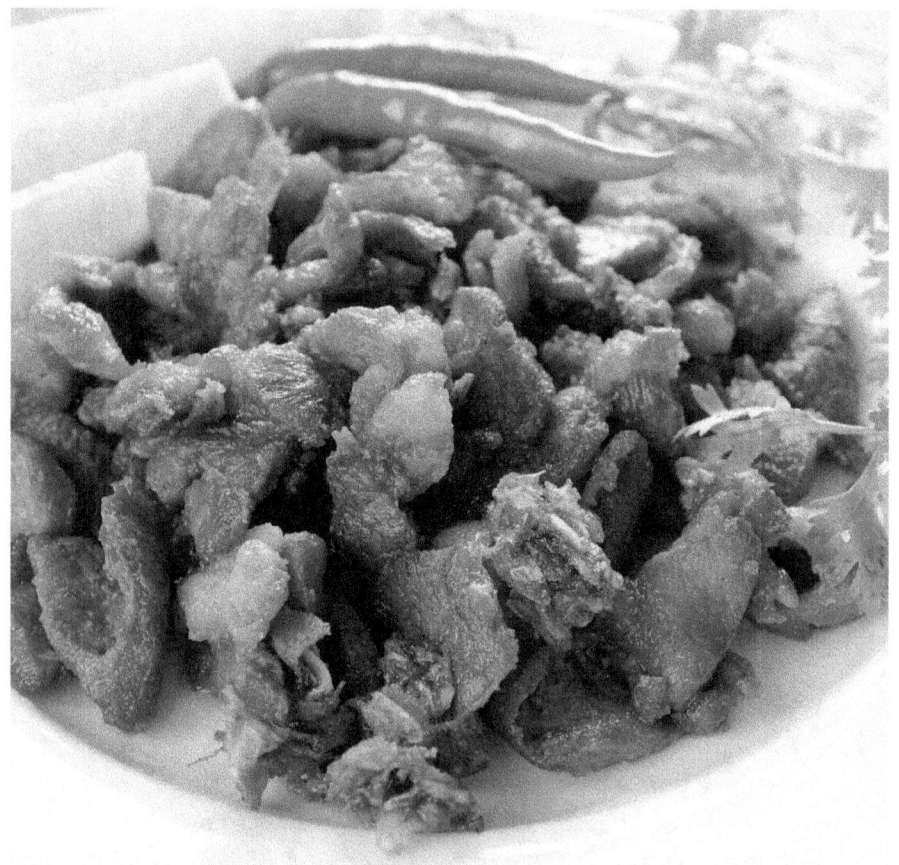

Servings Provided: 4

Time Required: 3 hours 40 minutes

What is Needed:

- Fresh pork tenderloin - lean cut (2 lb.)
- Soy sauce -shoyu - made from soy and wheat (.5 cup)
- Honey - strained/extracted (.33 cup)
- Ketchup (.33 cup)
- Brown sugar (.33 cup)
- Hoisin sauce - ready-to-serve (2 tbsp.)
- Rice wine (.25 cup)
- Red food coloring (.5 tsp.)
- Chinese Five-Spice Powder (1 tsp.)

Preparation Method:

1. Cut the pork "with the grain" into strips 1.5-2-inches long, and toss it into a large resealable zipper-type baggie.
2. Whisk the soy sauce, ketchup, honey, hoisin sauce, brown sugar, red food coloring, Chinese 5-spice, and rice wine in a saucepan using the med-low temperature setting. Simmer it until just combined and slightly warm (2-3 min.). Pour the marinade into the bag with the pork, pushing the air from the bag, and zip it closed. Toss the bag several times to cover all pork pieces.
3. Pop the pork in the fridge for two hours or overnight.
4. Warm the outdoor grill using the med-high temperature setting and lightly grease the grate.
5. Transfer the pork from marinade, shaking it to remove excess juices. Discard the marinade.
6. Grill the pork for 20 minutes. Place a container of water onto the grill and continue cooking, turning the pork until cooked thoroughly or about one hour. It's ready when the internal temp reaches 145° Fahrenheit.

Chinese Pork Dumplings

Servings Provided: 5/50 dumplings

Time Required: 1 hour 20 minutes

What is Needed:

- Soy sauce made from wheat & soy - shoyu (.5 cup)
- White rice vinegar CBT (1 tbsp.)
- Chinese chive - kucai - raw (1 tbsp.)
- Dried sesame seeds - whole (1 tbsp.)
- Sriracha sauce/Chili puree sauce w/Garlic CBT (1 tsp.)
- Freshly ground pork - raw (1 lb.)
- Garlic (3 cloves)
- Egg - whole (1)
- Kucai - Chinese chive - raw (2 tbsp.)

Preparation Method:

1. Combine ½ cup of the soy sauce, rice vinegar, sesame seeds, one tablespoon of chives, and the chile sauce in a small mixing container. Set it to the side for now.
2. Mix the pork, minced garlic, egg, two tablespoons of chives, soy sauce, sesame oil, and ginger in a large mixing container until thoroughly combined.
3. Lightly flour a workspace. Place a dumpling wrapper onto it and spoon

about one tablespoon of the filling in the center.
4. Wet the edge with a little water and crimp it together, forming small pleats to seal the dumpling. Repeat the process with the rest of the dumpling wrappers and filling.
5. Warm one to two tablespoons of oil in a large skillet using the med-high temperature setting. Arrange eight to ten dumplings in the pan and cook until browned (2 min. per side).
6. Pour in one cup of water, place a lid on the pot, and simmer until the pork is thoroughly cooked and the dumplings are tender (5 min.).
7. Continue the process until all dumplings are prepared. Serve with the soy sauce mixture for dipping.

Chop Suey

Servings Provided: 6

Time Required: 51 minutes

What is Needed:

- Fresh pork tenderloin (1 lb.)
- Wheat flour, all-purpose, white, enriched, bleached (.25 cup)
- Oil - soybean, salad or cooking (2 tbsp.)
- Bok choy - raw (2 cups)
- Celery - fresh (1 cup)
- Sweet red bell peppers (1 cup)

- Mushrooms (1 cup)
- Water chestnuts, Chinese, canned - solids & liquids (8 oz. can)
- Garlic (2 fresh cloves)
- Swanson Clear Chicken Broth CAM (.25 cup)
- Shoyu sauce (.25 cup)
- Cornstarch (1 tbsp.)
- Fleischmann's Cooking Sherry II (1 tbsp.)
- Ground ginger (.5 tsp.)

Preparation Method:

1. Use a sharp knife to discard the fat from the pork and slice it into one-inch pieces. Combine the flour and pork in a resealable bag, seal, and shake it thoroughly to cover.
2. Warm one tablespoon oil in a large skillet using the med-high heat setting. Add the trimmed pork and cook for three minutes or until browned. Transfer it to a container and keep it warm.
3. Pour the rest of the oil in the pan to heat. Add the celery, bok choy, mushrooms, red pepper, garlic, and water chestnuts. Stir-fry them for three minutes.
4. Thoroughly whisk the chicken broth, soy sauce, cornstarch, sherry, and ginger in a mixing container.
5. Combine the pork and broth mixture in a skillet, and cook for one minute or until thickened.

Easy Moo Shu Pork

Servings Provided: 6

Time Required: 1 hour 20 minutes

What is Needed:

- *Shoyu* - Soy sauce made from soy + wheat (2 tbsp.)
- Sesame oil (1 tbsp.)
- Garlic (1 tsp.)
- Fresh ginger root (1 tbsp.)
- Pork tenderloin (.75 lb.)
- Oil - soybean - salad or cooking (2 tbsp.)
- Chinese cabbage (pe-tsai) (2 cups)
- Carrots (1 raw)
- Salt (1 pinch)

Preparation Method:

1. Whisk the sesame oil, soy sauce, garlic and ginger in a bowl until the marinade is smooth. Dump it into a resealable plastic bag and add the pork. Cover it using the marinade, squeeze out any excess air, and seal the bag. Marinate in the fridge for a minimum of one hour to overnight.
2. Warm vegetable oil in a wok/large skillet using the medium temperature setting. Rinse and add the cabbage and diced carrot. Simmer the mixture for one to two minutes.
3. Push the cabbage mixture aside and add pork with marinade to the center of the skillet. Cook and stir until the pork is thoroughly cooked (3-4 min.).
4. Scoot the cabbage into the center of the skillet and continue to cook it for another minute or two. Adjust the flavor with a portion of pepper and salt to your liking.

Peking Pork Chops - Slow-Cooked

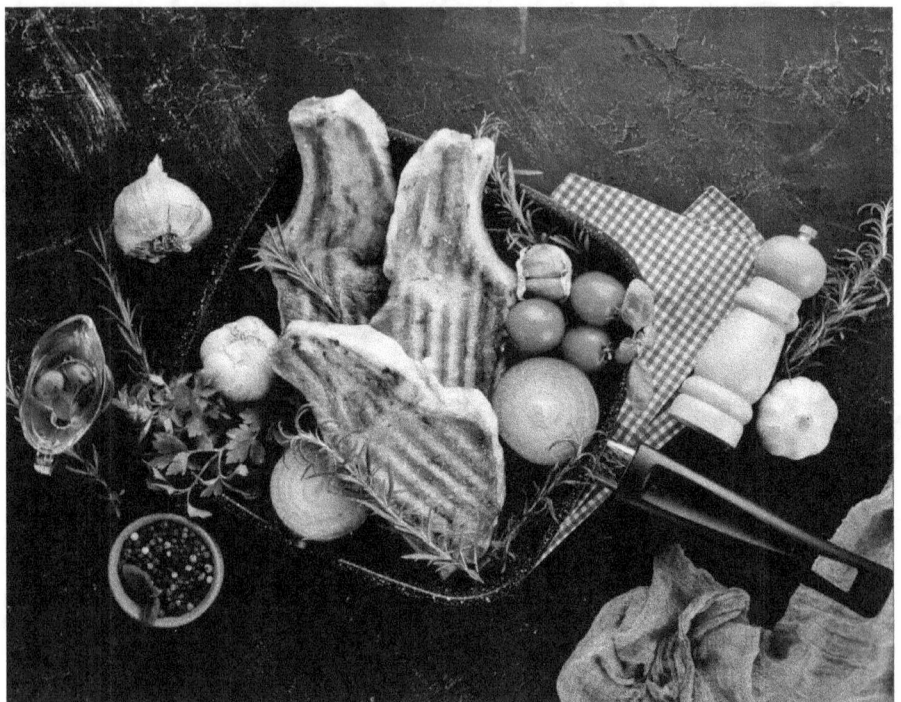

Servings Provided: 6

Time Required: 6 hours 15 minutes

What is Needed:

- Pork chops - top loin (6 boneless)
- Brown sugars (.25 cup)
- Ground ginger (1 tsp.)

- Shoyu soy sauce (.5 cup)
- Ketchup (.25 cup)
- Garlic (1 clove)
- Salt (as desired)

Preparation Method:

1. Use a sharp knife to remove the fat from the chops and toss them into the cooker.
2. Whisk the sugar, soy sauce, ginger, garlic, pepper, and salt. Dump it over the meat
3. Securely close the lid and set the timer for four to six hours.
4. Serve when it's tender with a dusting of salt and pepper as desired.

Chapter 5: Other Chinese Dishes

Crispy Tofu With Sweet & Sour Sauce

Servings Provided: 4

Time Required: 45 minutes

What is Needed:

The Sauce:

- Cornstarch (2 tsp.) + Water (2 tsp.)
- Garlic (2 minced cloves)
- Freshly grated ginger (.5 tsp.)
- Chili pepper flakes (.25 tsp.)
- Vegetable oil (2 tsp.)
- Water (.5 cup)
- Unseasoned rice vinegar (.33 cup)
- Agave nectar (.5 cup)
- Low-sodium soy sauce (2 tbsp.)
- Tomato paste (2 tbsp.)
- Sea salt (.25 tsp.)
The Tofu & Batter:

- Medium/firm tofu (1 brick)
- For Frying: Vegetable oil (3 cups)
- Cornstarch (1 tbsp.)
- Brown rice flour (1 cup)
- Ground pepper (.25 tsp.)
- Sea salt (.5 tsp.)
- Garlic powder (.5 tsp.)
- Cold soda water (1 cup)

Preparation Method:

1. Drain the brick of tofu and chop it into bite-sized cubes. Continue to drain the cubes on a layer of paper towels to remove the excess water. Press it often while you prepare the sauce.
2. Mix water with the cornstarch in a cup and set it aside for now.
3. Warm two teaspoons of vegetable oil using the med-low temperature setting. Mince and add the ginger, garlic, and chili pepper flakes. Stir for 30 seconds to one minute until fragrant.
4. Whisk in the rest of the sauce ingredients using the medium setting until it's bubbly. Whisk in the cornstarch mixture.
5. Whisk the sauce often for 10-12 minutes until slightly thickened. Transfer the pan to a cool burner while you prepare the crispy tofu.
6. Warm three cups of oil in an electric skillet or pan to reach 375° Fahrenheit.
7. Mix the batter by combining the rice flour, cornstarch, sea salt, garlic powder, and ground pepper in a mixing container.
8. When the pan is hot, stir in the soda water to the flour mixture and mix well.
9. Use your hands to coat three to four cubes of tofu and gently place them into the oil. Fry them for 2-2.5 minutes.
10. Remove the tofu using a slotted spoon and place them onto a layer of paper towels to absorb the excess fat. Repeat the process with the rest of the tofu cubes.
11. Warm the sauce if needed. In two to three batches, you can coat the crispy tofu with sauce by adding a portion of the sauce to a large bowl and tossing the crispy tofu cubes until coated evenly. Serve to your liking with veggies or rice.

Shiitake & Scallion Lo Mein

Servings Provided: 8

Time Required: 40 minutes

What is Needed:

- Lo mein noodles (1 lb.)
- Snow peas (.25 lb.)
- Mirin (.25 cup)
- Soy sauce (.25 cup)
- Toasted sesame oil (2 tsp.)
- Canola oil (3 tbsp.)
- Shiitake mushrooms (1 lb.)
- Scallions (6)
- Fresh ginger (1 tbsp.)
- Water (2 tbsp.)
- Cilantro (2 tbsp.)

Preparation Method:

1. Slice the snow peas diagonally into halves. Remove the stems and thinly slice the caps of the mushrooms. Cut the scallions into one-inch lengths. Mince the ginger and chop the cilantro.
2. Prepare a large pot of boiling salted water. Cook the noodles until tender, adding in the snow peas for the last two minutes of the cooking cycle. Rinse and drain the noodles and snow peas in a colander using

cold water until cooled.
3. Whisk the soy sauce with the sesame oil and mirin.
4. Prep a deep skillet to warm two tablespoons of the canola oil until shimmering using the high-temperature setting. Add the shiitake and cook it, undisturbed, until browned (5 min.).
5. Add the rest of the canola oil, scallions, and ginger. Stir-fry until the scallions softened (3 min.).
6. Add the water into the pan and simmer using moderate heat, scraping up the browned bits from the bottom of the pan for about a minute or so.
7. Mix in the snow peas, noodles, and soy sauce mixture. Simmer while tossing the noodles until they are thoroughly heated (2 min.).
8. Sprinkle using the cilantro and transfer it onto banana leaf cones or bowls to serve.

PART IV

Chapter 1: Tasty Breakfast Options

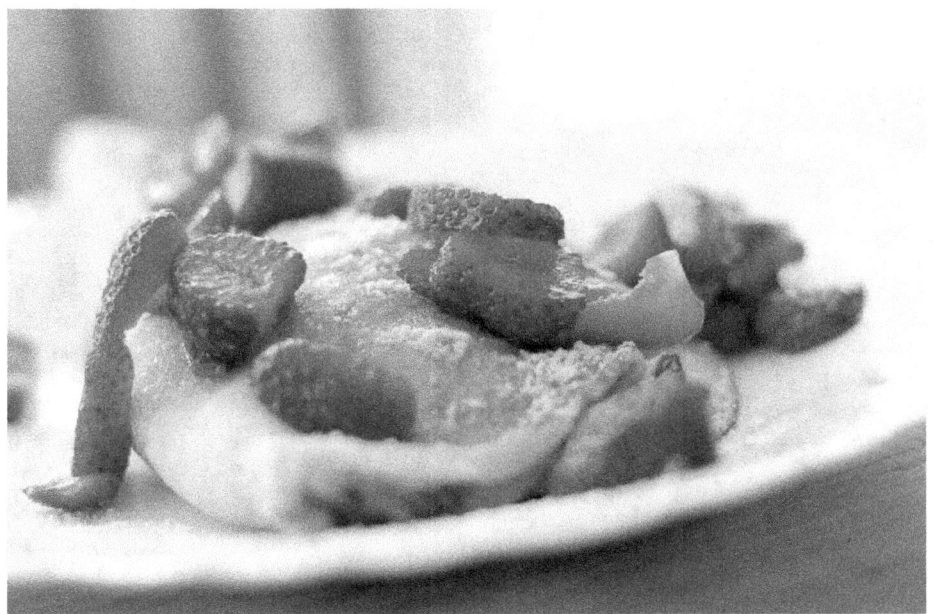

French Crepe

Servings Provided: 8

Time Required: 20 minutes

What is Needed:

The Crepes:

- Eggs (2)
- Melted butter (.25 cup)
- Sugar (2.5 tbsp.)
- A-P flour (.5 cup)

- Milk (.5 cup)
- Water (.125 cup)
- Vanilla (.5 tsp.)
- Dash (tiny dash)

The Filling:

- Powdered sugar (2-4 tbsp./as desired)
- Heavy whipping cream (1 cup)
- Vanilla extract (.5 tsp.)
- Freshly sliced strawberries
- Also Needed: **Non-stick - 6-inch skillet**

Preparation Method:

1. Prepare the crepes. Whisk all the fixings except the flour.
2. Fold in the flour - a little bit at a time - whisking just until the flour is incorporated.
3. Let the crepe batter rest for ten minutes. Whisk again before using it.
4. Grease the skillet with unsalted butter and warm it using the medium-temperature setting.
5. Pour about two to three tablespoons of batter into the pan - while tipping the pan from side to side to get the mixture spreading over the pan.
6. Cook each side of the crepe for half a minute before gently loosening the edges with a large spatula. If it lifts, it's ready to be flipped. If not, cook it for another 10-15 seconds and try again. Gently lift the crepe out of the pan, then flip over into the pan and cook the other side for another 10-15 seconds; remove to cool.
7. Prepare the filling. Use a hand/stand mixer to beat the heavy whipping

cream until soft peaks form. Add in the powdered sugar and vanilla. Continue mixing until stiff peaks form.
8. Spread a layer of cream over each crepe, sliced strawberries, and roll the crepe as you would a wrap.

French Omelette

Servings Provided: 1

Time Required: 15 minutes

What is Needed:

- Milk (1 tbsp.)
- Egg (1)
- Basil (1 tbsp.)
- Chives (1 tbsp.)
- Tarragon (.5 tbsp.)
- Salt and pepper (a pinch of each)
- Olive oil (as needed for the pan)
- Sundried tomato (1 thinly sliced - oil drained)
- Crumbled goat cheese (1 tbsp.)

Preparation Method:

1. Chop the basil, tarragon, and chives.
2. Whisk the milk, egg, salt, and pepper in a small mixing container. Add

half of the fresh herbs and gently stir to combine.

3. Add one tablespoon of olive oil to a small pan. Warm the oil using medium heat as you swirl it around the pan so that it coats the entire bottom of the pan and a little bit along the sides of the pan.

4. Dump the egg mixture into the pan. Swirl the pan so that the egg batter goes to the edges of the pan. Use a rubber spatula to gently push the egg batter to the edges of the pan.

5. Once the egg batter looks set on the bottom and is starting to bubble up a bit, lift the pan while tilting it to one side to slide the egg onto an awaiting using a large spatula. Flip the egg onto its other side into the pan and place it back on the burner using low heat.

6. Toss the crumbled cheese and tomato slices into the center of the omelet. Gently fold one side of the egg over, folding one more time - over itself (into thirds).

7. Serve promptly, garnished with the remaining fresh herbs.

Chapter 2: Delicious Salads

Traditional French Country Salad With Lemon Dijon Vinaigrette

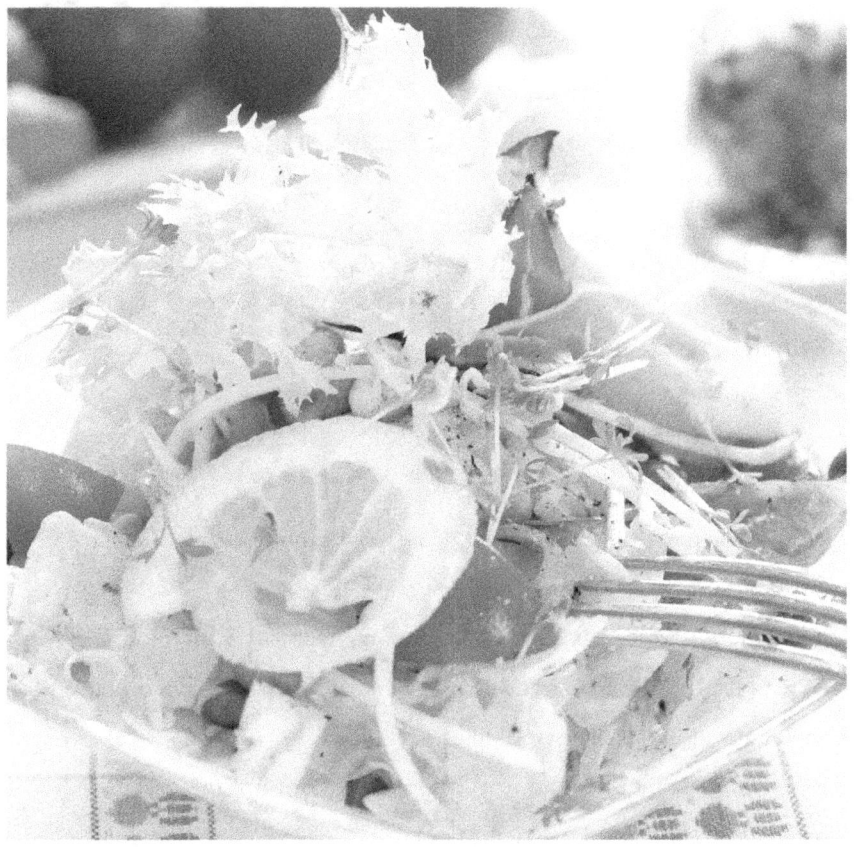

Servings Provided: 4

Time Required: 20 minutes

What is Needed:

- Arugula (5 oz. bag)
- Asparagus (.5 lb.)
- Olive oil (as desired)
- Sea salt (as desired)
- Sliced cooked beets (.5 cup)
- Whole walnuts or pecans, toasted (.5 cup)
- Crumbled goat cheese (.25 cup)
  The Vinaigrette:

- Balsamic vinegar (3 tbsp.)
- Dijon mustard (2 tbsp.)
- Olive oil (2 tbsp.)
- Minced garlic cloves (2 small)
- Sea salt & black pepper (.5 tsp./to taste)
- Lemon & zest (half of 1 lemon)

Preparation Method:

1. Set the oven at 400° Fahrenheit. Prepare a baking tray with a piece of parchment baking paper.
2. Trim the tattered ends and cut the asparagus into 1.5-inch long pieces. Spread it onto the prepared baking sheet. Drizzle the olive oil over the asparagus along with a sprinkle of sea salt.
3. Roast the asparagus for four to five minutes or until the asparagus is tender but still has a bite. Let it cool.
4. Toss the arugula with the asparagus in a large bowl.
5. Prepare the dressing. Whisk all of the vinaigrette fixings in a small measuring cup.
6. Assemble the salad. Toss the salad with the vinaigrette until everything is lightly coated, and garnish it using sliced beets, toasted nuts, and

crumbled goat cheese.

Chapter 3: Soup

Classic French Onion Bistro Soup

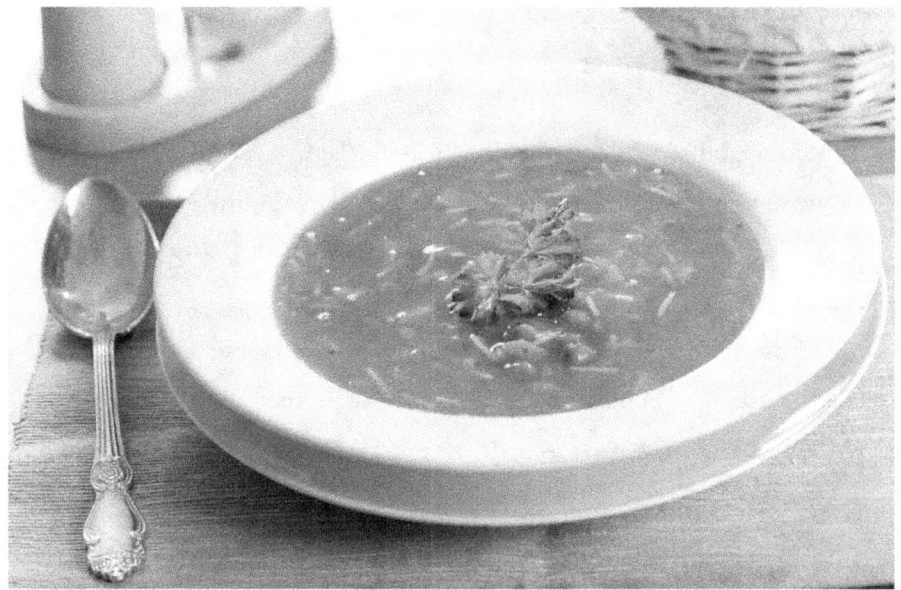

Servings Provided: 4

Time Required: 1.5 hours

What is Needed:

- Onions, (8 cups sliced/2 extra-large)
- Unsalted butter (1.5 tbsp.)
- Oil (1 tbsp.)
- Salt (.5 tsp.)
- Sugar (1 pinch)
- A-P flour (1.5 tbsp.)
- Low-sodium beef broth (4 cups)

- Pepper & salt (as desired)
- Sliced crusty French bread
- Gruyere cheese for the top/gruyere-cheddar mix (4 oz.)
- Also Needed: Oven-proof bowls (4)

Preparation Method:

1. Melt the butter with oil over low heat in a large pot or dutch oven. Slice the onions into crescent shapes and toss them into the pan. Place a lid on the pan and simmer them for about 15 minutes.
2. Slice the bread into ½-inch slices and toast them (set aside).
3. Adjust the stovetop temperature setting slightly higher and stir in the salt and sugar. Simmer with the lid off for another 40 to 45 minutes until onions have caramelized. Stir them occasionally throughout the duration.
4. Sprinkle the flour into the pot, stir, and simmer an additional three minutes.
5. Slowly add the broth into the pot, stirring as your pour. Season with a pinch of salt and pepper and cook for another 20 minutes until simmering and hot.
6. Warm the oven at 350° Fahrenheit.
7. Once the soup is ready, divide the soup into bowls. Place four to five baguette slices into each bowl. Top each bowl with grated cheese (.25 cup each dish).
8. Bake them until the cheese completely melts and serve promptly.

Fresh French Pea Soup

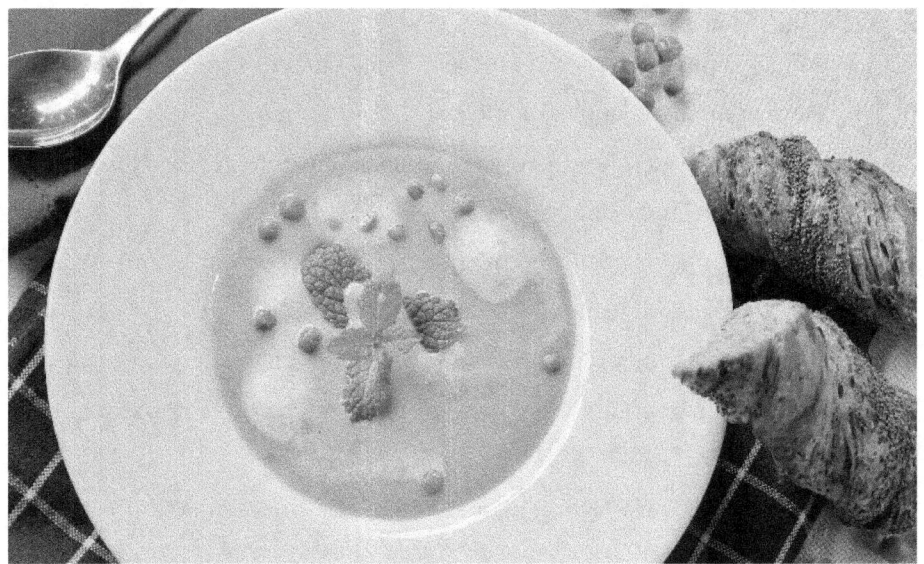

Servings Provided: 4

Time Required: 17 minutes

What is Needed:

- Butter with salt (2 tbsp.)
- Shallots (2 medium)
- Water (2 cups)
- Fresh green peas (3 cups)
- Table salt (.25 tsp.)

- Heavy whipping cream (3 tbsp.)

Preparation Method:

1. Prepare a heavy-bottomed saucepan (medium temp) to melt the butter. Sauté the shallots until soft and translucent (3 min.).
2. Pour in the water, peas, pepper, and salt. Adjust the temperature setting to med-high and bring to a boil.
3. Once boiling, lower the temperature setting to low, cover, and simmer until the peas are tender (12-18 min.).
4. Puree the peas in a food processor/blender in batches. Strain the pureed peas back into the saucepan, stir in the cream, and warm until it's piping hot.
5. Season to your liking with pepper and salt before serving.

Green Vegetable Soup

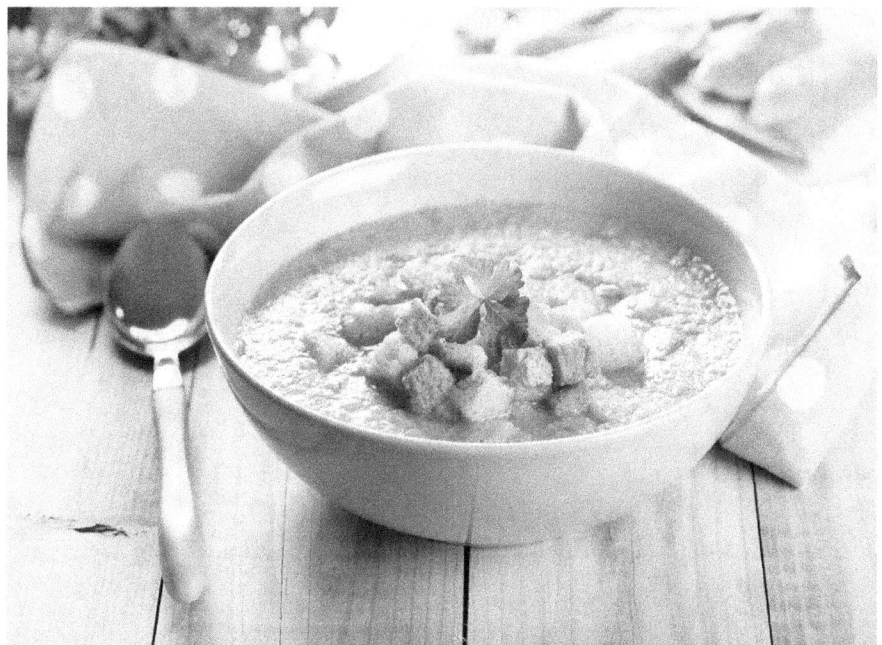

Servings Provided: 6

Time Required: 1 hour 40 minutes

What is Needed:

- Onions (2)
- Garlic (3 cloves)
- Butter, with salt (3 tbsp.)
- Swanson Clear Chicken Broth CAM (2 - 14.5 oz. cans)

- Water (4.5 cups)
- Carrots (3)
- Leeks (1)
- Spring onions/scallions - include tops & bulb (3)
- Habanero pepper (1 ½)
- Spinach (10 oz. bag)
- Watercress (1 bunch - raw)
- Table salt (1 tbsp.)
- Extra-virgin olive oil NOI (.25 cup)
- Red wine vinegar (50 Grain) NAK (.125 cup)

Preparation Method:

1. Warm a skillet using the med-high temperature setting. Sauté the minced garlic and onion (5 min.).
2. Add the water, chicken stock, spinach, carrots, green onions, leeks, habanero peppers, and watercress. Prepare it using a low-boil until the carrots are softened (30 min.). Remove the pan from the burner, and cool it for about half an hour.
3. When cooled, puree the soup in a food processor until smooth. Pour the mixture into the pot, and simmer using the low-temperature setting for 15 minutes.
4. Serve with a drizzle of olive oil and vinegar to your liking.

Chapter 4: Beef Options

Beef Bourguignon - Slow-Cooked

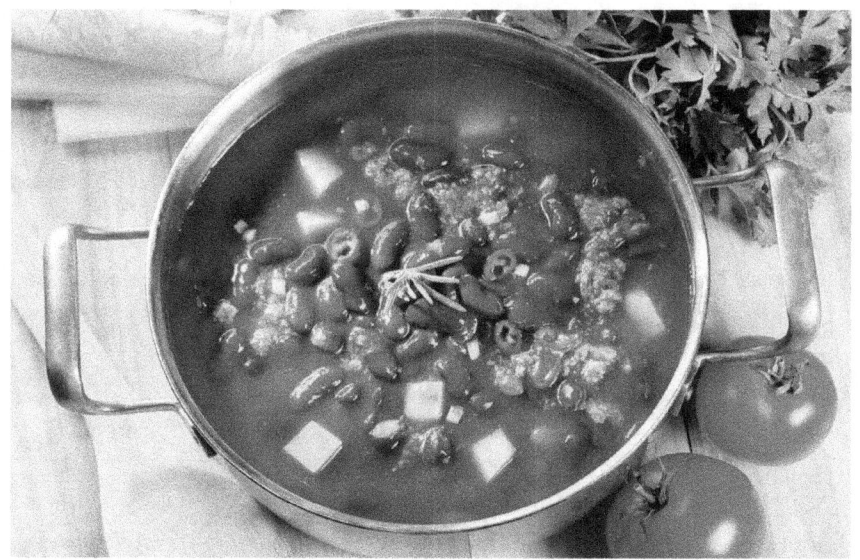

Servings Provided: 6

Time Required: 2.5 hours

What is Needed:

- Bacon (6 oz. - diced)
- Beef chuck (3 lb.)
- Large onion (1 chopped)
- Carrots (1)
- Garlic (2 minced cloves)
- A-P flour (3 tbsp.)
- Beef broth (1.5 cups)
- Red wine (¼ of a bottle)
- Salt (1 tsp.)

- Black pepper (1 pinch)
- Rosemary (1 sprig)
- Thyme (2 sprigs)
- Bay leaf (1)
- Olive oil (2 tbsp.)
- White mushrooms (7-8 thick slices)
- Pearl onions (10 oz.)
- For the Garnish: Fresh parsley

Preparation Method:

1. Warm a dutch oven or other large pot to cook the diced bacon using the med-high temperature setting. When it's nicely browned, transfer it to a paper-lined platter using a slotted spoon. Save the diced bacon for breakfast or a dish of mashed potatoes or just trash it.
2. Slice the beef into two-inch portions and toss it into the pot to brown each side. Remove the meat from the pan.
3. Chop and mix in the onion to sauté until it's translucent (5 min.). Mince and add the garlic to sauté for about half a minute.
4. Add the beef back into the pot and dust it with three tablespoons of flour. Stir the meat until the flour has been absorbed (1 min.).
5. Add in the beef broth and just enough red wine to almost fully immerse it in juices. Stir and add a teaspoon of pepper and salt as desired.
6. Tie the rosemary, thyme, and bay leaf together with a piece of kitchen twine, and drop the bouquet into the pot. Slice the carrots in half lengthwise, then cut into one-inch wide pieces, and add the carrots into the pot as well. Simmer them using the medium temperature setting. Cover the pot with a lid and adjust the temperature setting to med-low. Simmer the stew for about 2.2 to 3 hours until the beef is very tender.
7. Warm the olive oil in a large skillet using the med-low temperature setting. Add the sliced mushrooms and pearl onions, cooking until both are softened (7-8 min.). Set aside until ready to serve.
8. After the beef is ready, remove the herb packet.
9. Prepare a shallow bowl with the meat, sautéed mushrooms, pearl onions, and carrots. Add the sauce and garnish with a portion of chopped parsley

Entrecote Steak With Red Wine Sauce

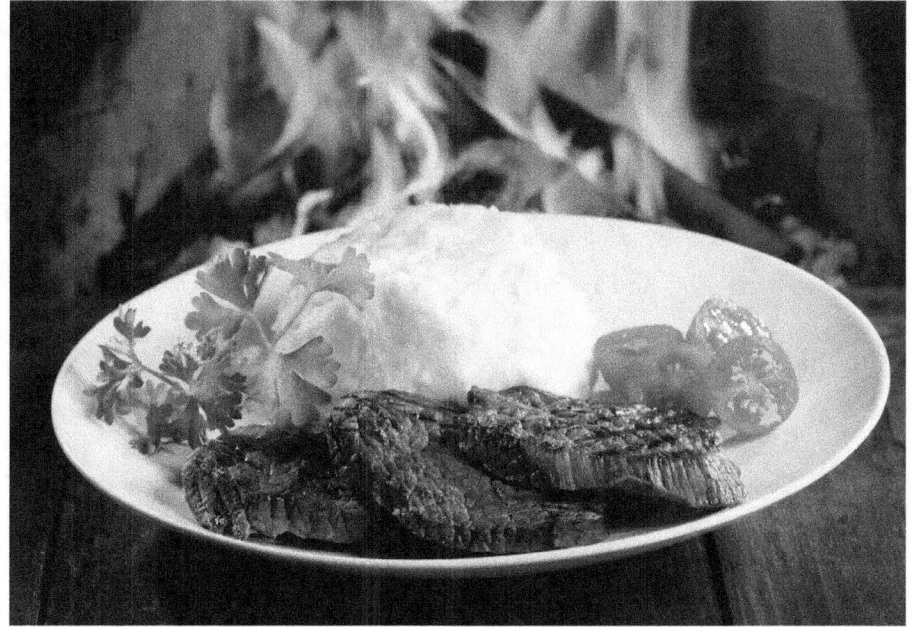

Servings Provided: 2

Time Required: 16 minutes

What is Needed:

- Rib-eye steaks (2 small)
- Black pepper & salt (as desired)
- Butter - unsalted (3 tbsp.)
- Shallot (1)
- Red wine (3 tbsp.)

- Beef stock (1/3 cup + 1 tbsp.)
- To Garnish: freshly chopped parsley

Preparation Method:

1. Generously sprinkle the steaks with pepper and salt.
2. Warm a cast-iron skillet using the high-temperature setting until it's 'smoking' hot. Add 1.5 tablespoons of butter to the pan, adjusting the setting to med-high.
3. Add the steaks to the hot buttered pan to cook for three minutes per side (medium doneness). Transfer the steaks to a platter for now.
4. Finely chop and add the shallot to the pan and sauté them for about a minute. Add the wine, and scrape the tasty browned bits with the juices from the bottom of the pan.
5. Reduce the temperature setting to medium, and stir in the beef stock. Simmer the mixture until the liquid has reduced by about half. Stir in the rest of the butter and prepare to serve it.
6. Use a sharp knife to slice the steaks at an angle and add the sauce. Garnish with a portion of fresh parsley.
7. Serve with your favorite side dish (ex. mashed potatoes, veggies, or french fries).

Pan-Seared Steak au Poivre

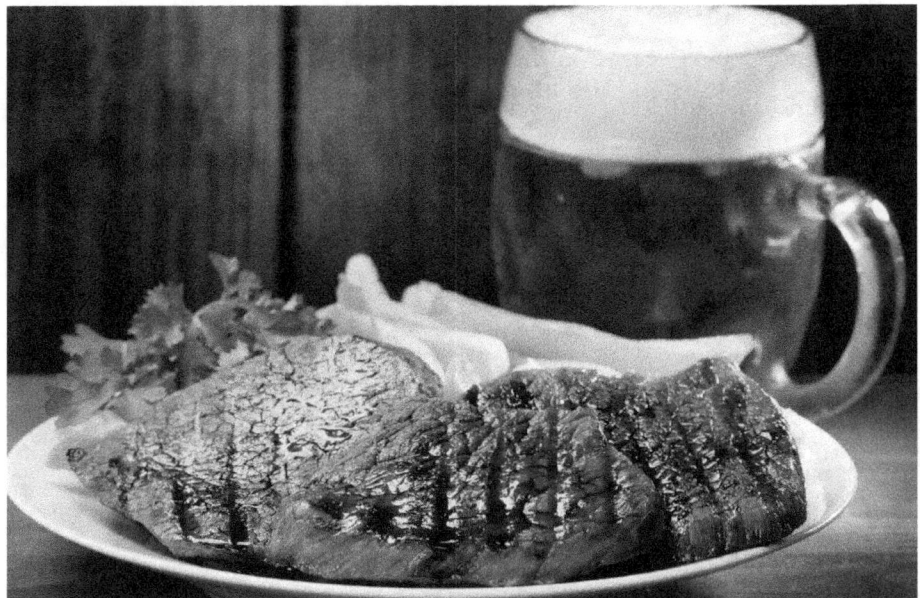

Servings Provided: 4

Time Required: 30 minutes

What is Needed:

- Filet mignons (4 small 1-inch each)
- Black peppercorns - cracked (1 tbsp.)
- Beef broth (.5 cup)
- Olive oil (1 tbsp.)
- Optional: Cognac (.25 cup)
- Cubed butter (2 tbsp.)

Preparation Method:

1. Use a paper towel to pat dry each filet and dust with pepper.
2. Warm a heavy cast-iron skillet using the medium-high heat until it's 'smoking' hot.
3. Flip the steaks and cook until small drops of red juice come to the surface (5 min. for medium). Transfer to a platter and keep them warm until time to add them to the mixture.
4. Empty the broth into the skillet to heat using the high-temperature setting and scrape up any browned bits.
5. At this point, add in the cognac and boil for one to two minutes to burn off the alcohol.
6. Remove the skillet from the burner. Whisk in the butter one cube at a time until melted.
7. Pour the sauce over the steaks and serve.

Steak Diane

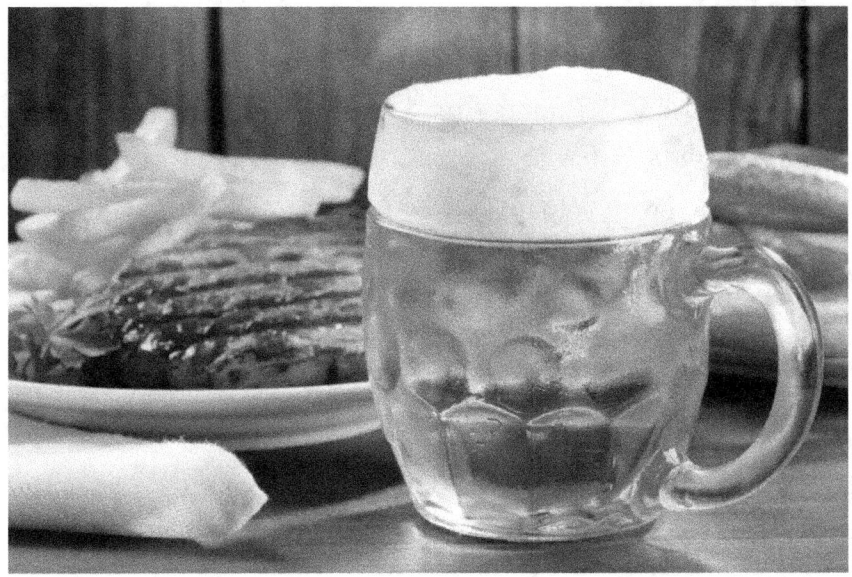

Servings Provided: 2

Time Required: 30 minutes

What is Needed:

- Jus De Veau Lie/Veal Demi-Glace-Pwd FD (.5 cup)
- Dijon Mustard NB (1 tbsp.)
- Worcestershire Sauce (2 tsp.)
- Tomato paste - salt added (1 tsp. - canned)
- Spices - pepper, red or cayenne (1 pinch)
  The Steaks:

- Soybean oil (2 tsp.)
- Beef tenderloin (2 - 8 oz. trimmed to ¼- inch thickness)
- Black pepper & kosher salt (as desired)
- Butter - no-salt (1 tbsp.)
- Shallots (3 tbsp.)
- Cognac (.25 cup)
- Heavy whipping cream (.25 cup)
- Chives (2 tsp.)

Preparation Method:

1. Generously sprinkle the steaks with salt. Wait for them to reach room temperature while you make the sauce.
2. Use the high-temperature setting to warm the oil. Once it reaches a smoking point, add the steaks, and dot them with a few chunks of butter.
3. Sear the meat (high temp) until brown on each side, two to three minutes on each side, keeping them on the rare side (internal temp of 125° Fahrenheit. Transfer steaks to a warm plate.
4. Toss the shallots into the skillet and sauté them until softened (2-3 min.).
5. Remove the skillet to a cool burner and add in the Cognac. Carefully ignite it using a fireplace lighter. After the alcohol burns off and the flames go out, return the skillet to the high setting and wait for it to boil. Simmer for a few minutes to reduce its volume slightly.
6. Add demi-glace mixture, cream, and any accumulated juices from the steak. Cook on high heat just until the sauce starts to thicken (3-5 min.).
7. Transfer the steaks back into the pan and adjust the temperature setting

to low. Gently simmer until meat is heated through and cooked to your desired level of doneness.
8. Serve on a heated plate with a generous portion of sauce. Sprinkle with chives to your liking and serve.

Chapter 5: Other Delicious French Classics

French Ham & Grilled Cheese Sandwich - Croque Monsieur

Servings Provided: 4

Time Required: 25 minutes

What is Needed:

- Sourdough toast (8 slices)
- Gruyere cheese (8 oz.)
- Black forest ham (8 slices)
- Bechamel sauce (1 recipe)
- Dijon mustard

The Sauce:

- Whole milk (1 cup)
- Unsalted butter (1 tbsp.)
- A-P flour (2 tbsp.)
- Pepper and salt (to your liking)

Preparation Method:

1. Make the sauce by warming the milk in a small saucepan using the med-low temperature setting until steam rises from the milk, but it has yet to boil. *Don't boil.*
2. Use another saucepan to melt the butter. Sift in the flour to create a bubbly, paste-like mixture. Slowly pour in hot milk, whisking it with a pinch of salt and pepper to your liking.
3. Stir the bechamel sauce using the low-temperature setting until it's thick enough to coat the back of a wooden spoon.
4. Set the oven using the broil function. Toast the bread slices and spread them with the mustard over half of the bread.
5. Prepare the sandwich using two slices of ham and shredded cheese on each. Top it using the ham with more shredded cheese.
6. Put the remaining bread slices over the ham and cheese to assemble the sandwiches. Spread about one to two tablespoons of bechamel sauce over the top of each sandwich. Sprinkle more shredded cheese on top of the bechamel.
7. Place the sandwiches on a baking tray and place the pan on the center oven rack until the cheese starts to melt.
8. Move the sandwiches to the top rack for about 30 seconds, removing when the cheese starts to obtain little golden spots.

Pork Chops With Mustard Sauce

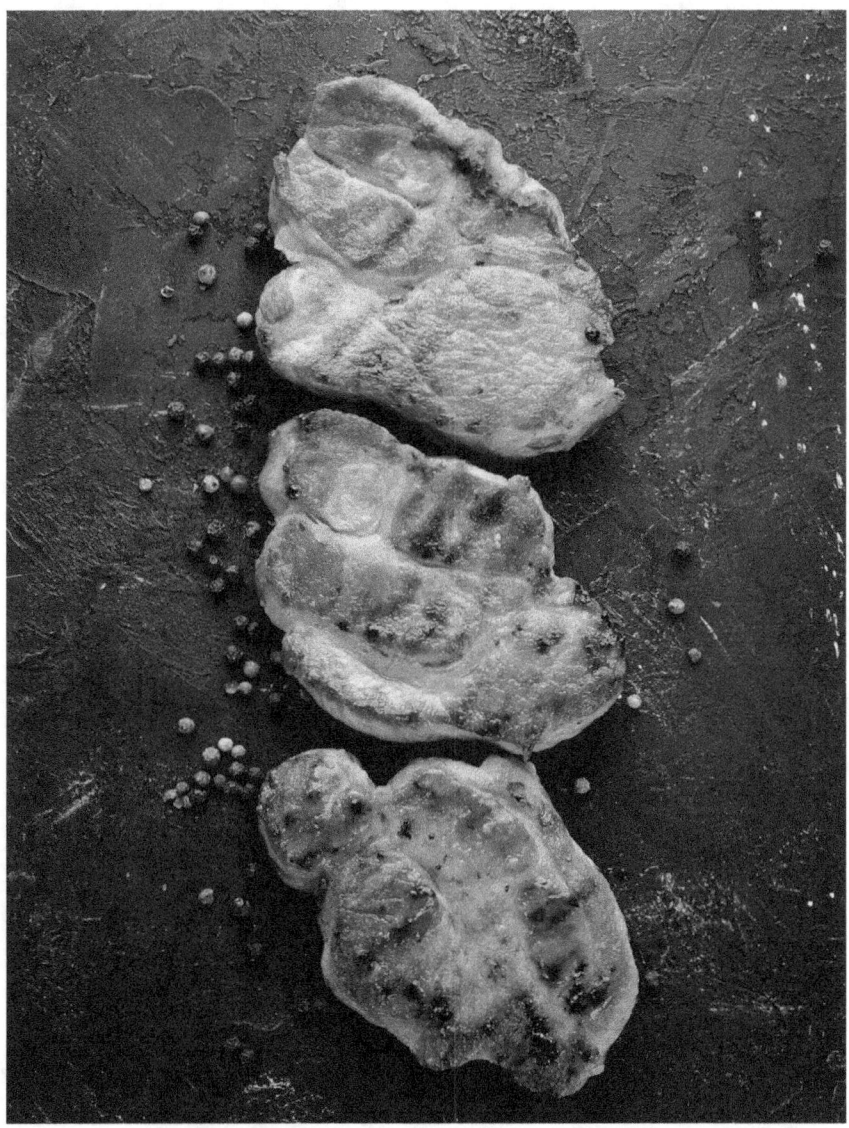

Servings Provided: 4

Time Required: 20 minutes

What is Needed:

- Olive oil (3 tbsp.)
- Boneless pork chops (4 - 1-inch or 1.5 lb.)
- Black pepper & kosher salt (.5 tsp. each/as desired)
- Finely chopped shallots (2)
- Dry white wine (.75 cup)
- Heavy cream (2 tbsp.)
- Dijon mustard (1 tbsp.)
- Freshly chopped tarragon (1 tbsp.)
- Torn frisée pieces (1 small head/4 cups)
- Lemon wedges (1)

Preparation Method:

1. Heat oven to 400° Fahrenheit.
2. Warm one tablespoon of the oil in a large skillet using the medium-high temperature setting.
3. Sprinkle the pork using pepper and salt. Let them cook and brown for two to three minutes per side.
4. Transfer the pork to a baking tray and roast until thoroughly cooked (5-7 min.).
5. Meanwhile, add the shallots and one tablespoon of the oil to the skillet and cook, often stirring, until softened (3-4 min.)
6. Add the wine to the skillet and simmer until reduced by half. Add the cream and simmer until the sauce just thickens. Stir in the mustard.
7. Top the pork with the sauce and tarragon. Drizzle the frisée with the remaining tablespoon of oil and serve with the lemon wedges.

Provencal Chicken Casserole

Servings Provided: 4

Time Required: 53 minutes

What is Needed:

- Olive oil (5 tbsp.)
- Chicken - broilers/fryers/breast - meat only (4 @ 6 oz.)
- Lemon juice (1 lemon)
- Table salt (1 pinch)
- Cherry tomatoes (1.5 cups)
- Onions - Spring/scallions - include tops & bulb (1 bunch)
- Swanson Clear Chicken Broth CAM (.5 cup)
- Brown mustard - prepared (2 tbsp.)
- Fresh rosemary (1.5 sprigs)
- Fresh thyme (half bunch)
- Cheese - gruyere (2 cups)

Preparation Method:

1. Pour three tablespoons of olive oil into a shallow platter and lay chicken breasts on top. Rub with lemon juice, salt, and pepper.
2. Warm two tablespoons of olive oil in a nonstick skillet using the med-high temperature function. Cook the chicken breasts until browned (4 min. per side).
3. Preheat the oven at 350° Fahrenheit. Grease a baking dish. Place

tomatoes and green onions in the baking dish and pour the chicken broth on top.

4. Whisk the mustard, rosemary, and thyme in a small bowl and brush onto chicken breasts. Arrange the chicken breasts on top of the vegetables in the baking dish. Cover with the Gruyere cheese.

5. Bake the casserole on the middle rack until the chicken juices run clear and are no longer pink in the center (30 min.). (You can test it using an instant-read thermometer inserted into the center for a reading of at least 165° Fahrenheit.)

White Wine Coq Au Vin

Servings Provided: 6

Time Required: 55 minutes

What is Needed:

- Chicken - thighs, breasts & drumsticks (8 pieces/3 lb.)
- Black pepper & kosher salt
- Unsalted butter (2 tbsp.)
- Sliced bacon (4 diced)

- Large sweet onion (1)
- Garlic (3 minced cloves)
- Cremini mushrooms (1 pint - sliced)
- Dry white wine (2 cups)
- Whole-grain mustard (1 tbsp.)
- Heavy cream (.5 cup)
- Freshly chopped parsley (.25 cup)

Preparation Method:

1. Season the chicken with pepper and salt. Melt the butter in a large skillet using the medium temperature setting.
2. Arrange the chicken in the skillet and cook until it's well browned (4 min. per side).
3. Transfer the chicken from the skillet and set it aside. Add the bacon to the skillet and cook until the fat begins to render (3 min.).
4. Dice and mix in the onion and sauté until it is translucent (5 min.). Add the garlic and mushrooms, and sauté until the mushrooms are tender (5-6 min.).
5. Add the browned chicken back to the skillet. Pour the wine into the skillet, stir in the mustard, and bring the mixture to a simmer using the med-low temperature function. Cover the skillet and simmer until the chicken is almost fully cooked (15-20 min.).
6. Uncover the skillet and add the cream. Simmer until the sauce thickens and the chicken is fully cooked (8-10 min.).
7. Garnish with parsley and serve immediately.

PART V

Are you worried that your hormones are not at their optimal levels? Here is a diet that will solve your problems.

Chapter 1: Health Benefits of the Hormone Diet

When it comes to getting healthy through weight loss, there's never any shortage of fitness crazes and diets that claim to have the secret to easy and sustainable weight loss. One of the latest diet plans that have come into the spotlight is the hormone diet, which claims that people often struggle to lose weight because of their hormones.

A hormone diet is a 3-step process that spans over six weeks and is designed to synchronize your hormones and promote a healthy body through detoxification, nutritional supplements, exercise, and diet. The diet controls what you eat and informs you about the correct time to eat to ensure maximum benefits to your hormones. Many books have been written on this topic with supporters of the diet assuring people that they can lose weight quickly and significantly through diet and exercise and reset or manipulate their hormones. Although the diet has a few variations, the central idea around each is that correcting the body's perceived hormonal imbalances is the key to losing weight.

The most important benefit of a hormone diet is that it takes a solid stance on improving overall health through weight loss and promoting regular exercise as well as natural, nutritious foods. Apart from that, it also focuses on adequate sleep, stress management, emotional health, and other healthy lifestyle habits that are all essential components that people should follow, whether it's a part of a diet or not. Including a water diet, it aims towards losing about twelve pounds in the 1st phase and 2 pounds a week after that.

Hormones have an essential role in the body's everyday processes, like helping bones grow, digesting food, etc. They act as "chemical messengers," instructing the cells to perform specific actions and are transported around the body through the bloodstream.

One of the very important food items to be included in the hormone diet is salmon. Salmon is rich in omega-3 fatty acids, Docosahexaenoic acid, and Eicosapentaenoic acid (EPA). It is rich in selenium too. These help to lower your blood pressure and also reduce the level of unhealthy cholesterol in the blood. These make you less prone to heart diseases. Salmon is a rich source of healthy fat. If consumed in sufficient amounts, it provides you energy and helps you get rid of unwanted body fat. Salmon is well-known for giving fantastic weight loss results as it has less saturated fat, unlike other protein sources. Salmon is packed with vitamins like vitamin-k, E, D, and A. These are extremely helpful for your eyes, bone joints, etc. These vitamins are also good for your brain, regulation of metabolic balance, and repairing your muscles. Salmon's vitamins and omega-3 fatty acids are amazing for sharpening your mind. It also improves your memory retention power. If you consume salmon, you are less likely to develop dementia or mental dis-functions. Salmon has anti-inflammatory properties and is low in omega-6 fatty acid content (which is pro-inflammatory in nature and is present in a huge amount in the modern diet). It promotes healthy skin and gives you radiant and glowing skin. It is good for the winter because it helps you to stay warm. It also provides lubrication to your joints because of the abundant presence of essential minerals and fatty acids in it. Apart from this, some other things to include in your diet are arugula, kale, ginger, avocado, carrots, and so on.

There are almost sixteen hormones that can influence weight. For example, the hormone leptin produced by your fat cells is considered a "satiety hormone," which makes you feel full by reducing your appetite. As a signaling hormone, it communicates with the part of your brain (hypothalamus) that controls food intake and appetite. Leptin informs the brain when there is enough fat in storage, and extra fat is not required. This helps prevent overeating. Individuals who are obese or overweight generally have very high levels of leptin in their blood. Research shows that the level of leptin in obese individuals was almost four times higher than that in individuals with normal weight.

Studies have found that fat hormones like leptin and adiponectin can promote long-term weight loss by reducing appetite and increasing metabolism. It is believed that both these fat hormones follow the same pathway in the brain to manage blood sugar (glucose) and body weight (Robert V. Considine, 1996).

Simply put, the hormone diet works by helping to create a calorie deficit through better nutritional habits and exercise, which ultimately results in weight loss. It's also essential to consult a doctor before following this detox diet or consuming any dietary supplements.

Chapter 2: Hormone-Rebalancing Smoothies

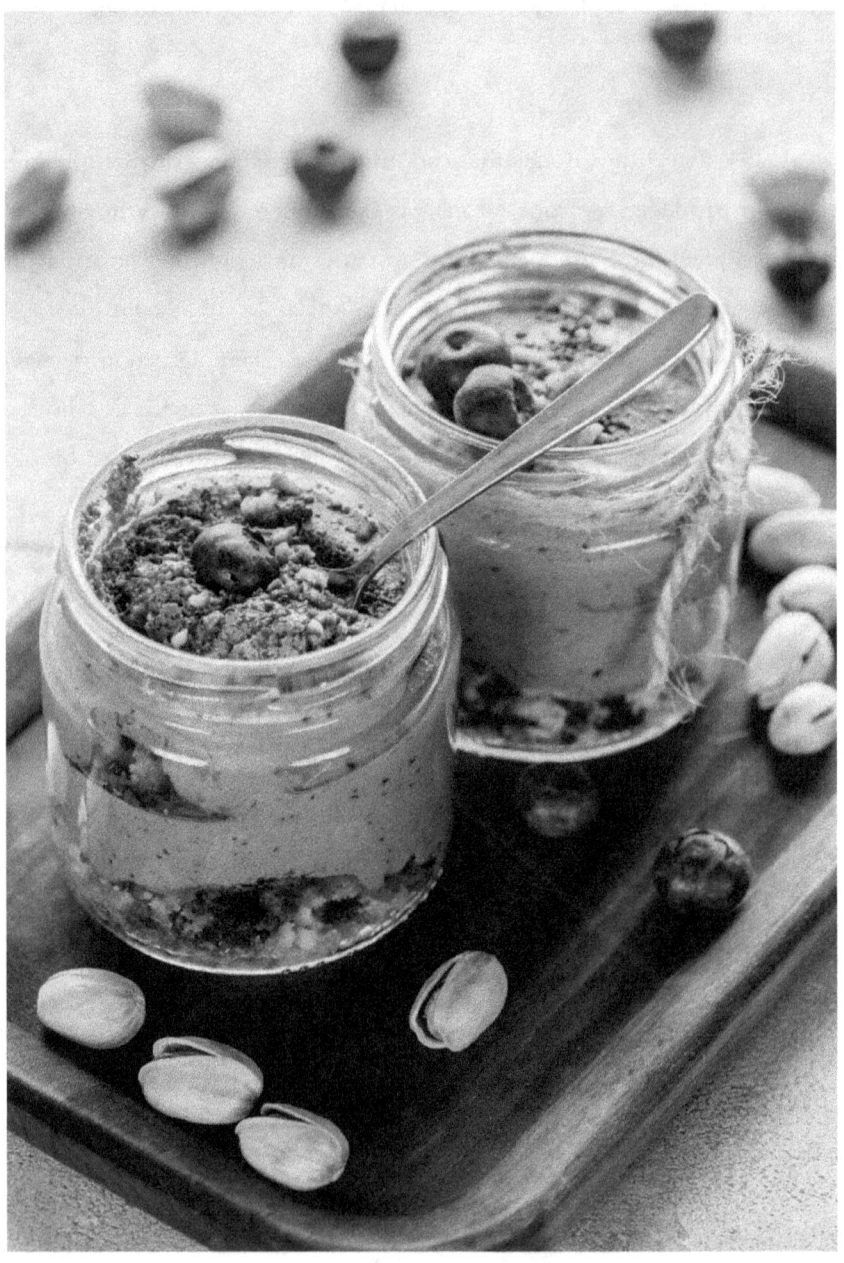

Estrogen Detox Smoothie

Total Prep & Cooking Time: 5 minutes

Yields: One glass

Nutrition Facts: Calories: 312 | Carbs: 47.9g | Protein: 18.6g | Fat: 8.5g | Fiber: 3g

Ingredients:

- Half a cup of hemp seeds
- Two kiwis (medium-sized)
- A quarter each of
    - Avocado (medium-sized)
    - Cucumber (medium-sized)
- Half a unit each of
    - Lemon (squeezed freshly)
    - Green apple
- One celery (medium-sized)
- A quarter cup of cilantro
- Two tbsps. of chis seeds
- Two cups of water (filtered)
- One tsp. of cacao nibs
- One tbsp. of coconut oil

Method:

1. Blend the ingredients all together to form a smoothie at high speed. The thickness can be adjusted according to your preference by adding more water to the mixture.

2. Serve and enjoy.

Dopamine Delight Smoothie

Total Prep Time: 10 minutes

Yields: One serving

Nutrition Facts: Calories: 383 | Carbs: 31g | Protein: 24g | Fat: 18.g | Fiber: 3g

Ingredients:

- Half a teaspoon of cinnamon (ground)
- Half a cup of peeled banana (the bananas must be frozen)
- One organic espresso, double shot (measuring half a cup)
- One tablespoon of chia seeds
- A three-fourth cup of soy milk (plain or vanilla-flavored)
- Protein powder, a serving (from the whey with the flavor of vanilla)

Method:

1. Fill in the bowl of your blender with all the ingredients (from the section of ingredients) except the whey protein powder and then proceed by switching to a high-speed blending option. Make sure it acquires a smooth consistency and then pour it out.

2. Now you may add the protein powder and give it another shot of blend until the whole things get incorporated, a bit of the goat cheese (already crumbled).

Breakfast Smoothie Bowl

Total Prep Time: 10 minutes

Yields: 2 servings

Nutrition Facts: Calories: 290 | Carbs: 53g | Protein: 6g | Fat: 8g | Fiber: 9g

Ingredients:

- One cup of thoroughly rinsed blueberries (fresh and ripe)
- A sundry of nuts and fruits for garnishing, which includes – strawberries, bananas (thinly sliced), peanuts (Spanish), kiwi (chopped), segments of tangerine, and raspberries.
- One cup of Greek yogurt

For the preparation of honey flax granola,

- Two tablespoons each of
    - Flaxseeds
    - Vegetable oil
- Oats (old-fashioned), approximately a cup
- One tablespoon of honey

Method:

1. Set your oven at a temperature of 350 degrees F.

2. Preparation of the smoothie: collect the diverse types of berries, wash them thoroughly, and then put them in the blender and turn it on. Make an even mixture out of it. Add some amount of the yogurt and blend it again to form a smooth texture.

3. For preparing the granola: Take a small-sized bowl and then drizzle a few drops oil in it. Then add the oats, flax, and honey to the oil, one by one, and mix it well. You are required to toss the bowl thoroughly to get the mixture well-coated with the poured oil. After you are done, place the oats mixture in a baking sheet evenly. Bake it for about twenty minutes. This mark will be enough to give the oats a beautiful tinge of golden brown. Allow it to cool.

4. Now you will require a shallow bowl to spoon in some yogurt, and this will be the first layer. Form a second layer with the various fruits and nuts and finally for the third layer, top with the granola.

5. Enjoy.

Notes:

- *Using frozen nuts and fruits in a warm-weather will get much to your relief.*

- *For a vegan smoothie bowl, sub the yogurt with coconut or almond yogurt.*

- *Give the pan a few strokes while baking the oats.*

Blueberry Detox Smoothie

Total Prep Time: Ten minutes

Yields: One serving

Nutrition Facts: Calories: 326 | Carbs: 65g | Protein: 4g | Fat: 8g | Fiber: 9g

Ingredients:

- One cup of wild blueberries (frozen)
- One banana (sliced into several pieces) frozen
- Orange juice (approximately half a cup)
- Cilantro leaves, fresh (approximately a measuring a small handful size)
- A quarter of an entire avocado
- A quarter cup of water

Method:

1. Add cilantro, avocado, water, blueberries, banana, and orange juice in the blender and then process.//
2. Make the ingredients integrated so well that they become smooth in their consistency.

Notes: *It is recommended that you add the potent herb, cilantro, or parsley in a small amount when consuming this smoothie for the first time, as it might trigger a mild headache. If you do not get a headache, you may add a bit more of the cilantro leaves.*

Maca Mango Smoothie

Total Prep & Cooking Time: 2 minutes

Yields: 2 servings

Nutrition Facts: Calories: 53 | Carbs: 13g | Protein: 1g | Fat: 3g | Fiber: 1.5g

Ingredients:

- One and a half cups each of
    - Fresh mango
    - Frozen mango
- One tablespoon each of
    - Ground flaxseed
    - Nut butter
- One teaspoon of ground turmeric
- Two teaspoons of maca root powder
- Three-quarter cups of nut milk
- One frozen banana

Method:

1. Blend all the ingredients together to get a smooth mixture.
2. Adjust consistency by adding nut milk.
3. Once done, divide into two glasses and enjoy!

Pituitary Relief Smoothie

Total Prep & Cooking Time: 5 minutes

Yields: 2 servings

Nutrition Facts: Calories: 174 | Carbs: 18.3g | Protein: 9.7g | Fat: 8.3g | Fiber: 14.4g

Ingredients:

- One teaspoon of coconut oil
- One fresh or frozen ripe banana
- One tablespoon of raw sesame seeds
- Two teaspoons each of
  - Chia seeds
  - Raw Maca powder
  - Raw Spirulina
- Two cups of water
- Two tablespoons of hulled hemp seeds

Method:

1. You have to use a blender to process this smoothie. Add the hulled hemp seeds, sesame seeds, and water in the blender and process them. Do it at high speed, and it will only require a minute. This will give you raw-milk like texture.

2. Then, add the following ingredients into it – coconut oil, banana, chia seeds, Maca, and Spirulina, and process the ingredients once again but this time on medium speed for another minute or so. Everything will become well incorporated.

3. You have to drink this smoothie on an empty stomach.

Notes: *In order to make the smoothie rich in antioxidants, you can add some fresh fruits like blueberries, kiwi, and raspberries.*

Chapter 2: Easy Breakfast Recipes

Scrambled Eggs With Feta and Tomatoes

Total Prep & Cooking Time: 10 minutes

Yields: One Plate

Nutrition Facts: Calories: 421 | Carbs: 8.6g | Protein: 20.3g | Fat: 35.1g | Fiber: 1.6g

Ingredients:

- One tbsp. each of
    - Olive oil (extra virgin)
    - Freshly chopped parsley, basil, dill or chives
- Half a cup of cherry tomatoes (each tomato sliced into half)
- Two ounces of crumbled feta cheese (approximately a quarter cup)
- Two eggs are beaten
- Two tbsp. of onion (diced)
- To taste:
    - Black pepper
    - Kosher salt

Method:

1. Keep the beaten eggs in a small-sized bowl and then season it with a pinch of pepper and salt. Set the bowl aside.

2. Use a nonstick skillet to proceed with the cooking. Pour two tbsp. of olive oil. Then add the diced onions. Stir over moderate heat and cook until softened. Make sure that the onions do not look brown. This process should get done by a minute.

3. Add half a cup of tomatoes to skillet and then continue to mix for about two minutes.

4. Now you may add the eggs. Using a spatula, gather the beaten eggs to the center by moving spatula all over the skillet.

5. The eggs will take an additional minute to get cooked. So after that mark, add the parsley or other herbs (if preferred) and feta cheese. Keep the eggs underdone as they will get cooked completely after they are served in the plate itself (from the residual heat). Therefore, cook the entire thing in the skillet for 30 seconds only.

6. Take a serving plate and transfer the eggs to it. Top with some sprinkled parsley and feta cheese, drizzled with some oil, and seasoned with some pepper and salt. These additions are optional and may vary as per your desire.

Smashed Avo and Quinoa

Total Prep & Cooking Time: 15 minutes

Yields: Six bowls

Nutrition Facts: Calories: 492 | Carbs: 67g | Protein: 15g | Fat: 20g | Fiber: 13g

Ingredients:

- One avocado skinned, cut into half, and then pitted
- A handful of cilantro or coriander
- Half a lemon (juiced)
- A quarter red onion (diced finely)
- One-eighth teaspoon of cayenne pepper
- To taste: Sea salt

For the Greens,

- One handful of kale
- One handful of soft herbs (basil, parsley or mint)
- One handful of chard or spinach
- For frying: butter or coconut oil

Serve with,

- One cup of quinoa (cooked)

Method:

1. You will require a frying pan to get this done. To it, add the coconut oil or butter (whichever you prefer) and add the greens. Toss them carefully and then sauté over moderate heat. Stop when they become soft.

2. Mix the onion, cayenne, avocado, cilantro, salt, lemon, and pepper to a bowl and mix them completely. The pepper and salt must be added according to the taste.

3. Add cooked quinoa to the tossed greens and heat altogether over low heat.

4. Take a serving plate and place the quinoa mixture and greens to it. Crown the whole thing with smashed avocado and then serve.

Hormone Balancing Granola

Total Prep & Cooking Time: 35 minutes

Yields: 8 servings

Nutrition Facts: Calories: 360 | Carbs: 19.8g | Protein: 5.1g | Fat: 28.8g | Fiber: 5.8g

Ingredients:

- One-third cup each of
    - Flaxseed meal
    - Pumpkin seeds
    - Seedless raisins
- Two teaspoons of cinnamon
- One teaspoon of vanilla extract
- Four tablespoons of maple syrup
- Five tablespoons of melted coconut oil
- A quarter cup of unsweetened coconut flakes
- Two-thirds cup each of
    - Chopped pecans
    - Chopped brazil nuts
- Two tablespoons of ground chia seeds

Method:

1. Set the temperature of the oven to 180 degrees F and preheat.

2. In a food processor, chop the pecans and the Brazil nuts. Then, mix these chopped nuts with coconut flakes, seeds, and other nuts present in the list of ingredients.

3. Add maple syrup, coconut oil, cinnamon, and vanilla extract in a separate bowl and combine well.

4. Now, take the wet ingredients and pour them into the dry ingredients. Mix thoroughly so that everything has become coated properly.

5. Place the prepared mixture in the oven for half an hour and cook.

6. Once done, cut into pieces and serve.

Chapter 3: Healthy Lunch Recipes

Easy Shakshuka

Total Prep & Cooking Time: 30 minutes

Yields: Six servings

Nutrition Facts: Calories: 154 | Carbs: 4.1g | Protein: 9g | Fat: 7.8g | Fiber: 0g

Ingredients:

- Olive oil (extra virgin)
- Two chopped green peppers
- One teaspoon each of
    - Paprika (sweet)
    - Coriander (ground)
- A pinch of red pepper (flakes)
- Half a cup of tomato sauce
- A quarter cup each of
    - Mint leaves (freshly chopped)
    - Parsley leaves (chopped freshly)
- One yellow onion, large-sized (chopped)
- Two cloves of garlic, chopped
- Half a teaspoon of cumin (ground)
- Six cups of chopped tomatoes (Vine-ripe)
- Six large-sized eggs
- To taste: Pepper and salt

Method:

1. You will require a large-sized skillet (made of cast iron). Pour three tablespoons of oil and heat it. After bringing the oil to boil, add the peppers, spices, onions, garlic, pepper, and salt. Stir time to time to cook the veggies for five minutes until they become softened.

2. After the vegetables become soft, add the chopped tomatoes and then tomato sauce. Cover the skillet and simmer for an additional fifteen minutes.

3. Now, you may remove the lid from the pan and then cook a touch more to thicken the consistency. At this point, you may adjust the taste.

4. Make six cavities within the tomato mixture and crack one egg each inside the cavities.

5. Cover the skillet after reducing the heat and allow it to cook so that the eggs settle into the cavities.

6. Keep track of the time and accordingly uncover the skillet and then add mint and parsley. Season with more black and red pepper according to your desire. Serve them warm with the sort of bread you wish.

Ginger Chicken

Total Prep & Cooking Time: 50 minutes

Yields: Six Servings

Nutrition Facts: Calories: 310 | Carbs: 6g | Protein: 37g | Fat: 16g | Fiber: 1g

Ingredients:

- A one-kilogram pack of chicken thighs (skinless and boneless)
- Four cloves of garlic (chopped finely)
- A fifteen-gram pack of coriander (fresh and chopped)
- Two tablespoons of sunflower oil
- One teaspoon each of
    - Turmeric (ground)
    - Chili powder (mild)
- A four hundred milliliter can of coconut milk (reduced-fat)
- One cube of chicken stock
- One ginger properly peeled and chopped finely (it should be of the size of a thumb)
- One lime, juiced
- Two medium-sized onions
- One red chili, sliced and the seeds removed (fresh)

Method:

1. Make the chicken thighs into three large chunks and marinate them with chili powder, garlic, coriander (half of the entire amount), ginger, oil (one tbsp.), and lime juice. Cover the bowl after stirring them well and then store it in the fridge until oven-ready.

2. Marinade the chicken and keep overnight for better flavor.

3. Chop the onions finely (it is going to be the simplest for preparing the curry) before dropping them into the food processor. Pour oil into the frying pan (large-sized) and heat it. Then add chopped onions and stir them thoroughly for eight minutes until the pieces become soft. Then pour the turmeric powder and stir for an additional minute.

4. Now add the chicken mixture and cook on high heat until you notice a change in its color. Pour the chicken stock, chili, and coconut milk and after covering the pan simmer for another twenty minutes. Sprinkle the left-over coriander leaves and then serve hot.

5. Enjoy.

Carrot and Miso Soup

Total Prep & Cooking Time: 1 hour

Yields: Four bowls of soup

Nutrition Facts: Calories: 76 | Carbs: 8.76g | Protein: 4.83g | Fat: 2.44g | Fiber: 1.5g

Ingredients:

- Two tbsps. of oil
- Garlic, minced (four cloves)
- One inch of garlic (grated)
- Three tbsps. of miso paste (white)
- One diced onion
- One pound of carrot (sliced thinly)
- Four cups of vegetable stock
- To taste: Pepper and Salt

For garnishing,

- Two scallions (sliced thinly)
- Chili pepper (seven spices)
- One nori roasted (make thin slivers)
- Sesame oil

Method:

1. Using a soup pot will be convenient to proceed with. Pour oil in a pot and then heat over a high flame. Now you may put garlic, carrot, and onion and sauté them thoroughly. Cook for about ten minutes so that the onions turn translucent.

2. Then add the ginger and vegetable stock. Mix them well and cook all together. Put the flame to simmer. Cover the pot while cooking to make the carrot tender. This will take another thirty minutes.

3. Put off the flame and puree the soup with the help of an immersion blender.

4. Use a small-sized bowl to whisk together a spoonful of the soup and the white miso paste. Stir until the paste dissolve and pour the mixture back to the pot.

5. Add pepper and salt if required.

6. Divide the soup among four bowls and enrich its feel by adding scallions, sesame oil, seven spices, and nori.

Arugula Salad

Total Prep & Cooking Time: 1 hour 10 minutes

Yields: Two bowls of salad

Nutrition Facts: Calories: 336.8 | Carbs: 30.6g | Protein: 7.7g | Fat: 22.2g | Fiber: 7.3g

Ingredients:

For the salad,

- Two medium-sized beets (boiled or roasted for about an hour), skinned and sliced into pieces that can easily be bitten
- Four tablespoons of goat cheese
- Approximately 2.5 oz. of baby arugula (fresh)
- A quarter cup of walnuts (chopped roughly before toasting)

For the dressing,

- Three tablespoons of olive oil (extra virgin)
- A quarter tsp. each of
    - Mustard powder (dried)
    - Pepper
- Half a tsp. each of
    - Salt
    - Sugar

- One and a half tablespoons of lemon juice

Method:

1. For preparing the vinaigrette, place all the ingredients (listed in the dressing ingredients section) in a jar and then shake them to emulsify. At this stage, before starting with the process of emulsification, you may add or remove the ingredients as per your liking.

2. Get the salad assembled (again depending upon the taste you want to give it), add a fistful of arugula leaves, place some chopped beets (after they have been cooked), and finally the toasted walnuts (already chopped).

3. Drizzle vinaigrette over the salad and enjoy.

Notes:

- *Coat the beets with oil (olive), roll them up in an aluminum foil, and then roast the beets at a temperature of 400 degrees F.*

- *And for boiling the beets, immerse them in water after transferring to a pot and simmer them for 45 minutes.*

Kale Soup

Total Prep & Cooking Time: 55 minutes

Yields: 8 servings

Nutrition Facts: Calories: 277.3 | Carbs: 50.9g | Protein: 9.6g | Fat: 4.5g | Fiber: 10.3g

Ingredients:

- Two tbsps. of dried parsley
- One tbsp. of Italian seasoning
- Salt and pepper
- Thirty oz. of drained cannellini beans
- Six peeled and cubed white potatoes
- Fifteen ounces of diced tomatoes
- Six vegetable Bouillon cubes
- Eight cups of water
- One bunch of kale (with chopped leaves and stems removed)
- Two tbsps. of chopped garlic
- One chopped yellow onion
- Two tbsps. of olive oil

Method:

1. At first, take a large soup pot, add in some olive oil, and heat it.
2. Add garlic and onion. Cook them until soft.
3. Then stir in the kale and cook for about two minutes, until wilted.
4. Pour the water and add the beans, potatoes, tomatoes, vegetable bouillon, parsley, and the Italian seasoning.
5. On medium heat, simmer the soup for about twenty-five minutes, until the potatoes are cooked through.
6. Finally, do the seasoning with salt and pepper according to your taste.

Roasted Sardines

Total Prep & Cooking Time: 25 minutes

Yields: 4 servings

Nutrition Facts: Calories: 418 | Carbs: 2.6g | Protein: 41g | Fat: 27.2g | Fiber: 0.8g

Ingredients:

- 3.5 oz. of cherry tomatoes (cut them in halves)
- One medium-sized red onion (chopped finely)
- Two tablespoons each of
    - Chopped parsley
    - Extra-virgin olive oil
- One clove of garlic (halved)
- Eight units of fresh sardines (gutted and cleaned, heads should be cleaned)
- A quarter teaspoon of chili flakes
- One teaspoon of toasted cumin seeds
- Half a lemon (zested and juiced)

Method:

1. Set the temperature of the oven to 180 degrees C and preheat. Take a roasting tray and grease it lightly.

2. Take a bowl and add the tomatoes and onions in it. Add the lemon juice too and toss the veggies in the lemon juice. Now, add the zest, olive oil, chili, cumin, garlic, and parsley and toss everything once again.

3. Use pepper and salt to season the mixture. The cavity of the sardines has to be filled. Use some of the tomato and onion mixture for this purpose. Once done, place the sardines on the prepared roasting tray. Take the remaining mixture and scatter it over the sardines.

4. Roast the sardines for about 10-15 minutes, and by the end of this, they should be cooked thoroughly.

5. Serve and enjoy!

Chapter 4: Tasty Dinner Recipes

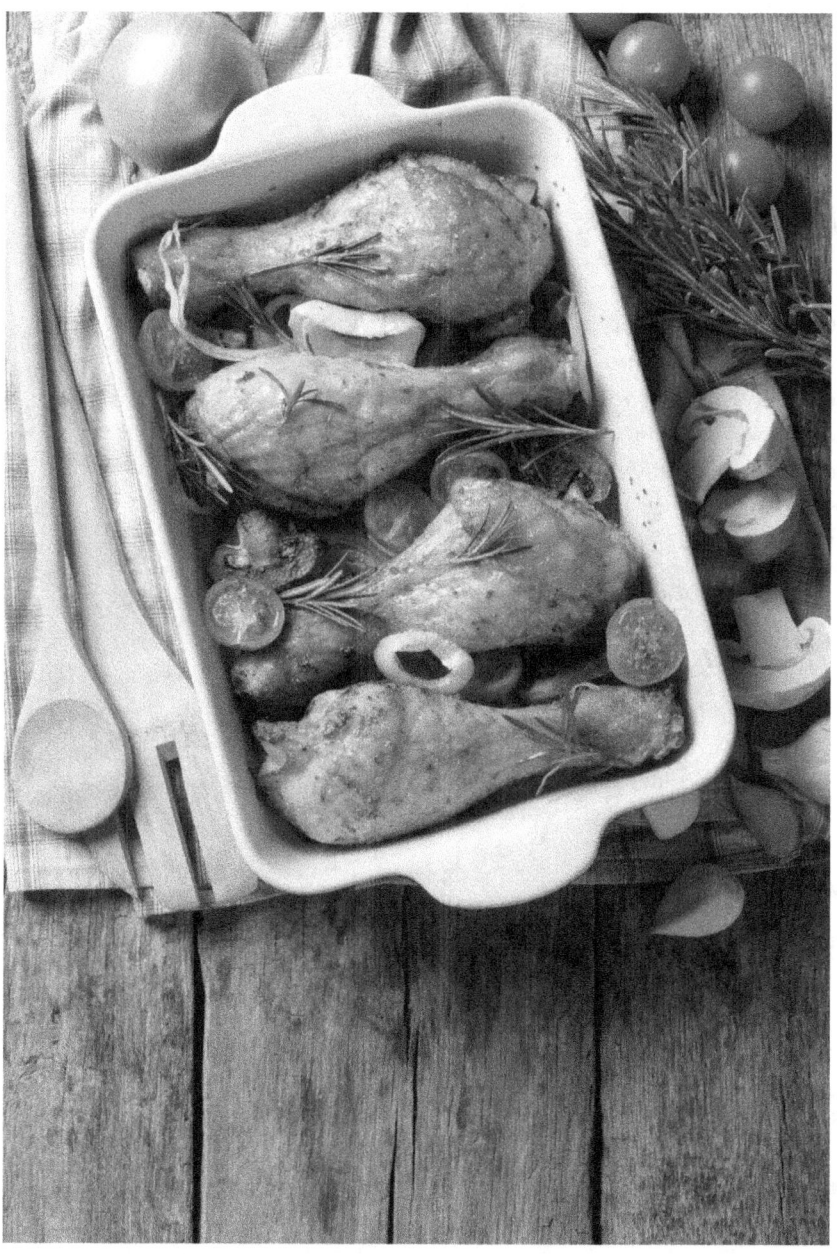

Rosemary Chicken

Total Prep & Cooking Time: 50 minutes

Yields: 4 servings

Nutrition Facts: Calories: 232 | Carbs: 3.9g | Protein: 26.7g | Fat: 11.6g | Fiber: 0.3g

Ingredients:

- Four chicken breast halves (skinless and boneless)
- One-eighth tsp. kosher salt
- One-fourth tsp. ground black pepper
- One and a half tbsps. of lemon juice
- One and a half tbsps. of Dijon mustard
- Two tbsps. of freshly minced rosemary
- Three tbsps. of olive oil
- Eight minced garlic cloves

Method

1. At first, preheat a grill to medium-high heat. The grate needs to be lightly oiled.

2. Take a bowl and add lemon juice, mustard, rosemary, olive oil, garlic, salt, and ground black pepper. Whisk them together.

3. Take a resealable plastic bag and place the chicken breasts in it. Over the chicken, pour the garlic mixture (reserve one-eighth cup of it).

4. Seal the bag and start massaging the marinade gently into the chicken. Allow it to stand for about thirty minutes at room temperature.

5. Then on the preheated grill, place the chicken and cook for about four minutes.

6. Flip the chicken and baste it with the marinade reserved and then cook for about five minutes, until thoroughly cooked.

Finally, cover it with a foil and allow it to rest for about 2 minutes before you serve them.

Corned Beef and Cabbage

Total Prep & Cooking Time: 2 hours 35 minutes

Yields: 5 servings

Nutrition Facts: Calories: 868.8 | Carbs: 75.8g | Protein: 50.2g | Fat: 41.5g | Fiber: 14g

Ingredients:

- One big cabbage head (cut it into small wedges)
- Five peeled carrots (chopped into three-inch pieces)
- Ten red potatoes (small)
- Three pounds of corned beef brisket (along with the packet of spice)

Method:

1. At first, in a Dutch oven or a large pot, place the corned beef, and cover it with water. Then add in the spices from the packet of spices that came along with the beef. Cover the pot, bring it to a boil, and finally reduce it to a simmer. Allow it to simmer for about 2 hours and 30 minutes or until tender.

2. Add carrots and whole potatoes, and cook them until the vegetables are tender. Add the cabbage wedges and cook for another fifteen minutes. Then finally remove the meat and allow it to rest for fifteen minutes.

3. Take a bowl, place the vegetables in it, and cover it. Add broth (which is reserved in the pot) as much as you want. Then finally cut the meat against the grain.

Roasted Parsnips and Carrots

Total Prep & Cooking Time: 1 hour

Yields: 4 servings

Nutrition Facts: Calories: 112 | Carbs: 27g | Protein: 2g | Fat: 1g | Fiber: 7g

Ingredients:

- Two tbsps. of freshly minced parsley or dill
- One and a half tsp. of freshly ground black pepper
- One tbsp. kosher salt
- Three tbsps. of olive oil
- One pound of unpeeled carrots
- Two pounds of peeled parsnips

Method:

1. At first, preheat your oven to 425 degrees.
2. If the carrots and parsnips are thick, then cut them into halves lengthwise.
3. Then, slice each of them diagonally into one inch thick slices. Don't cut them too small because the vegetables will anyway shrink while you cook them.
4. Take a sheet pan, and place the cut vegetables on it.
5. Then add some olive oil, pepper, salt, and toss them nicely.
6. Roast them for about twenty to forty minutes (the roasting time depends on the size of the vegetables), accompanied by occasional tossing. Continue to roast until the carrots and parsnips become tender.
7. Finally, sprinkle some dill and serve.

Herbed Salmon

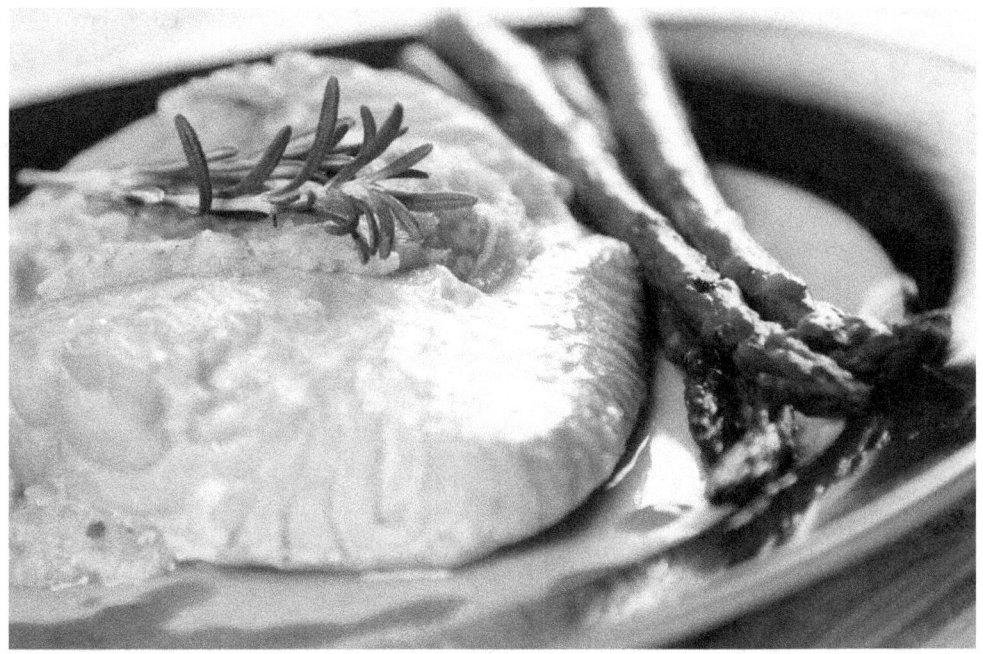

Total Prep & Cooking Time: 30 minutes

Yields: 4 servings

Nutrition Facts: Calories: 301 | Carbs: 1g | Protein: 29g | Fat: 19g | Fiber: 0g

Ingredients:

- Half a tsp. of dried thyme or two tsps. of freshly minced thyme
- Half a tsp. of pepper

- Three-fourth tsp. of salt
- One tbsp. of olive oil
- One tbsp. freshly minced rosemary or one tsp. of crushed dried rosemary.
- Four minced cloves of garlic
- Four (six ounces) fillets of salmon

Method:

1. At first, preheat your oven to 425 degrees.
2. Take a 15 by 10 by 1 inch baking pan and grease it.
3. Place the salmon on it while keeping the skin side down.
4. Combine the garlic cloves, rosemary, thyme, salt, and pepper. Spread it evenly over the salmon fillets.
5. Roast them for about fifteen to eighteen minutes until they reach your desired doneness.

Chipotle Cauliflower Tacos

Total Prep & Cooking Time: 30 minutes

Yields: 8 servings

Nutrition Facts: Calories: 440 | Carbs: 51.6g | Protein: 10.1g | Fat: 24g | Fiber: 9g

Ingredients:

For the tacos,

- Four tablespoons of avocado oil
- One head of cauliflower (large-sized, chopped into bite-sized florets)
- One cup of cilantro (freshly chopped)
- One tablespoon each of
    - Fresh lime juice
    - Maple syrup or honey
- Two tsps. of chipotle adobo sauce
- Cracked black pepper
- One teaspoon of salt
- 4-8 units of garlic cloves (freshly minced)

For the Chipotle Aioli,

- A quarter cup of chipotle adobo sauce
- Half a cup each of
    - Sour cream
    - Clean mayo

One teaspoon of sea salt

Two cloves of garlic (minced)

For serving,

- Almond flour tortillas
- Guacamole
- Almond ricotta cheese
- Sliced tomatoes, radish, and cabbage

Method:

1. Set the temperature of the oven to 425 degrees F. Now, use parchment paper to line a pan. Take the bite-sized florets of the cauliflower and spread them evenly on the pan. Use 2-4 tbsps. of avocado oil, pepper, salt, and minced garlic and drizzle it on the pan.

2. Roast the cauliflower for half an hour at 425 degrees F and halfway through the process, flip the florets.

3. When you are roasting the cauliflower, take the rest of the ingredients of the cauliflower and mix them in a bowl. Once everything has been properly incorporated, set the mixture aside.

4. Now, take another bowl and in it, add the ingredients of the chipotle aioli. Mix them and set the bowl aside.

5. If you have any other taco fixings, get them ready.

6. Once the cauliflower is ready, toss the florets in the chipotle sauce.

7. Serve the cauliflower in tortillas along with fixings of your choice and the chipotle aioli.

PART VI

Chapter 1: What is The Freestyle Way?

As you begin your journey using the Freestyle techniques, you will learn it utilizes the elements of calories in and calories out. The point system assigns specific points based on the nutritional and calorie content. Your activity level also influences how the points are assigned to offset against the food points.

One excellent online resource to discover your points is available at "healthyweightforum.org/eng/calculators/ww-points-allowed/" The information involved includes your gender, age, activity level, weight, height, and how many pounds you want to lose. The math is calculated for you to show how many points you can consume on your meal plan daily.

For example, a 65-year old woman who has a sedentary lifestyle, is 5'1" tall, 174 lbs. who wants to lose 10 pounds is allowed 24 points for the first 2 weeks and 23 points for the next 3 weeks.

All you need to do is add the points for additional optional or toppings that are not included in the recipe. Each food added to the product will possibly raise the content of fat or sugar. Proteins are calculated into the equation to help lower the points.

The goal is to get you on the right track of choosing leaner proteins and eating more fruits and vegetables with each meal. By increasing these food items, you are lowering the unhealthy fats and consuming less sugar. You will be surprised by many of the foods that contain -0- points. It's hard to believe they are diet-friendly foods!

Use your enclosed 21-day plan as a guideline to get your body in tune with the new way of eating healthier. It won't take long before you are inspired. Your family and friends will surely enjoy the tastier techniques used for food preparation. You will also love all of the new zero foods!

Zero Point Fruits

Enjoy most fruits in moderation - only because the calories can add up quickly. The only exceptions to the rule are plantains and avocados. Consider this as you prepare your smoothie, if you add any additional fruits - be sure to consider any possible points involved. This includes frozen or fresh fruit, as well as jarred or canned. Just remember to choose the ones packaged without added sugar.

Zero Point Vegetables

Many veggies are -0- points on the new Freestyle plan. However, as you prepare your meal, be sure to take into accounts the oil and butter used as you make the vegetables. Enjoy canned, fresh or frozen mushy peas, potatoes, parsnips, cassava, yuca, yams, sweet potatoes, and olives - without additional fats, oil, or sugars.

Zero Point Spices & Other Condiments

You can choose from many items including low-sugar condiments and spices. For example, enjoy items such as fresh or rubs, vinegar, broth, dried spices, hot sauce, mustard, salsa, and capers.

Remember, the points consumed will also depend on the amount you are using in your recipe. They may be zero points for a small serving, but collectively, as they are used in the recipe, they may contain more points.

Other Foods To Enjoy Freestyle

- Boneless & skinless chicken breast and turkey
- Ground lean chicken and turkey
- Thinly sliced deli chicken or turkey breast
- All shellfish and fish (excluding smoked or dried fish)
- Canned fish packed in brine or water
- Regular and smoked tofu
- Eggs
- Plain soy yogurt
- Plain Greek yogurt
- Fresh – frozen - canned beans and lentils that are packed without oil or sugar (Ex. Lentils, pinto beans, split peas, chickpeas, black beans, kidney beans, soybeans, and more)

Chapter 2: Breakfast Favourites

No matter what you are craving, just remember, breakfast is considered the most important meal of the day. So, enjoy each one of these selections as you adjust to your new way of meal preparation!

Baked Omelet

Freestyle Points: 2

Yields: 4 Servings

Ingredients:

- Egg whites – 3
- Large eggs - 3
- Greek yogurt - plain fat-free – 2 tbsp.
- Pepper - .25 tsp.
- Salt - .125 tsp.
- Onion - .25 cup
- Bell peppers - .25 cup
- Grated parmesan cheese - .25 cup
- Cubed ham - .5 cup
- Broccoli florets – 1 cup
- Baby spinach leaves – 2 cups
- For the Garnish: Green onion – 1
- Also Needed: -10-inch skillet

Preparation Method:

1. Warm up the temperature setting in the oven to 400°F.
2. Chop the veggies. Whip the yogurt, eggs, pepper, and salt until frothy using a hand mixer.

3. Warm up the skillet using the med-high setting and spray with oil to prevent sticking. Add the broccoli, peppers, ham, and onions. Lower the temperature to the medium heat setting. Continue cooking for approximately five minutes.
4. Toss in the spinach and continue cooking until wilted. Blend in the green onions and add the mixed eggs. Sprinkle with the parmesan.
5. Cook 10 minutes on the stovetop. Move it to the oven for 10 to 15 additional minutes until the eggs are done and set.
6. Garnish with a few green onions and parmesan cheese before serving.

Banana Roll-Ups

Freestyle Points:2

Yields: 1 Serving

Ingredients:

- Whole wheat bread – low-cal – 1 slice
- Medium peeled banana - .5 of 1
- Salt-free chunky peanut butter - 1.5 tsp.

Preparation Method:

1. Use a rolling pin or wine bottle as a substitute to flatten the bread.
2. Apply the peanut butter to one side of the bread. Add the banana.
3. Roll it up and slice into 3-4 segments.
4. Enjoy any time.

Broccoli Cheddar Egg Muffins

Freestyle Points: 2

Yields: 6 Servings

Ingredients:

- Egg whites - 4
- Whole eggs - 8
- Dijon mustard - .5 tbsp. - optional
- Broccoli – 2 cups **
- Shredded cheddar cheese - .75 cups
- Pepper and salt – to your liking
- Diced green onions - 2

** Use either fresh and steamed or defrosted and frozen broccoli.

Preparation Method:

1. Warm up the oven to 350°F. Prepare 6 muffin tins with paper liners or cooking spray.
2. Whisk all of the eggs, salt, pepper, and mustard. Blend in the green onions, broccoli, and cheese.
3. Divide up the batter and bake for 12-14 minutes.
4. Serve when they are puffy and thoroughly cooked.

Cinnamon-Apple French Toast

Freestyle Points: 4

Yields: 4 Servings

Ingredients:

- Liquid egg whites – 1.33 cups
- 1% milk – 1 cup
- Eggs – 4
- Cinnamon – 2 tsp.
- Apples – 2
- Slices of low-calorie bread – 8
- Also Needed: 9 x 13 casserole dish

Preparation Method:

1. Peel and dice the apples. Grease the baking dish with cooking spray. Prepare the oven temperature to 350°F.
2. Using a microwavable dish to combine and cook the cinnamon and apples for three minutes.
3. Line the baking dish with bread slices and a layer of cooked apples.
4. Whisk the egg whites and milk. Pour over the bread. Bake 45 minutes. Serve and enjoy with your favorite toppings.

Country Cottage Pancakes

Freestyle Points: 3

Yields: 4 Servings

Ingredients:

- Low-fat cottage cheese – 1 cup
- Medium eggs – 8
- Coconut flour – 4 tbsp.
- Bicarb of soda - .5 tsp.
- Almond flour – 4 tbsp.
- Grated zest of lemon – 1 tsp.
- Kosher salt – A pinch
- Vanilla essence - .5 tsp.
- Sweetened almond milk – 4 tbsp.

Preparation Method:

1. In a blender; combine all of the fixings – excluding the almond milk for now. Blitz until smooth.
2. Lightly spritz a skillet with cooking oil spray. Warm it up using medium-high temperature setting.
3. Prepare in four batches – one at a time. Flip only once, when the pancakes start bubbling. Continue cooking and serve immediately.

Egg & Sausage Muffins

Freestyle Points: 1

Yields: 20 Servings

Ingredients:

- Lean turkey breakfast sausage – 1 lb.
- Liquid egg whites – 3 cups
- Minced cloves of garlic - 2
- Green chilis – 4 oz. – 1 can - mild or hot
- Small chopped onion - 1
- Hash browns – 3 cups
- Black pepper – to your liking
- Sea salt – 1.5 tsp.

Preparation Method:

1. Warm up the oven to 375°F. Prepare 20 muffin tins with some cooking spray.
2. Cook the sausage on the stovetop using the med-high heat setting. As it breaks apart, stir in the onions, garlic, and chilies. Remove when the onions have softened.
3. Prepare the same skillet with a spritz of cooking spray. Toss in the hash browns, salt, and pepper the way you like it. Simmer 3-4 minutes. Fold in the eggs and combine well.
4. Dump the prepared batter into the tins. Bake 15-18 minutes. Check the centers for doneness using the toothpick test.

Egg & Veggie Scramble

Freestyle Points: 1

Yields: 6 Servings

Ingredients:

- Extra-virgin olive oil – 1.5 tbsp.
- Diced tomato - 1
- Large eggs - 6
- Baby spinach – 3 cups
- Minced garlic clove - 1
- Red or purple diced onion - .5 of 1
- Black pepper and Kosher salt – 1 tsp. of each
- 2% sharp cheddar cheese - .5 cup

Preparation Method:

1. Whisk the eggs, pepper, and salt.
2. Warm up the olive oil in a skillet. Toss in the spinach, tomato, onions, and garlic. Simmer until done or about 5-7 minutes.
3. Pour in the eggs and simmer 3-4 minutes – stirring occasionally. When set, remove from the burner and add the cheese on top. Serve and enjoy.

Hard-Boiled Eggs in the Instant Pot

Freestyle Points: -0-

Yields: Varies

Ingredients:

- Water – 1 cup
- Eggs - your choice in a single layer

Preparation Method:

1. Measure out the water and add to the pot. Gently add the eggs to the rack basket. Close the lid and set the timer for 3-5 minutes (high-pressure).
2. Natural release the pressure for 5 minutes and quick release the remainder of the built-up steam pressure.
3. Arrange the eggs in a cold-water dish to cool. A few ice cubes will speed the process. Wait 5-10 minutes before peeling.

Muffin Tin Eggs

Freestyle Points: 1

Yields: 6 Servings

Ingredients

- Eggs – 1 dozen
- Fat-free ground turkey breast - .5 lb.
- Diced green bell pepper – 1
- Steak seasoning – ex. Montreal Blend – 1 tsp.
- Red pepper flakes - .25 tsp.
- Black pepper and salt - .5 tsp. each
- Sage - .5 tsp.
- Marjoram - .25 tsp.
- Also Needed: -12-cup muffin tin

Preparation Method:

1. Set the oven temperature to 350°F. Prepare the muffin tin with cooking spray.
2. Spray the skillet and add the turkey, pepper flakes, black pepper, marjoram, salt, and sage. Cook for 7-10 minutes. Stir often to prevent sticking.
3. In a large mixing container, combine the steak seasoning and eggs - mixing well (2-3 min.) until fluffy. Blend in the diced pepper.
4. Once the turkey mixture is done, spoon into the tins and add the egg mixture. Fill about 3/4 full and bake for 30 minutes in the hot oven.

Tropical Breakfast Pie

Freestyle Points: 5

Yields: 4 Servings

Ingredients:

- Refrigerated biscuit dough – 7.5 oz.
- Unsweetened shredded coconut – 2 tbsp.
- Granulated sugar - .5 tsp.
- Fresh pineapple – 1 cup
- Also Needed: 8-inch-square casserole dish

Preparation Method:

1. Warm up the oven in advance to 350°F.
2. Lightly coat the casserole dish with a splash of cooking spray. Break apart the dough into 10 portions and slice into quarters.
3. Load a Ziploc-type bag with the sugar and coconut. Shake well and add the dough bits. Shake gently, but well to coat.
4. Place the biscuits into the dish and garnish with the diced pineapple.
1. Place in the preheated oven. Bake for 25 minutes.

Zucchini Noodles & Poached Eggs – Instant Pot

Freestyle Points: 4

Yields: 3 Servings

Ingredients for the Noodles:

- Olive oil – 1 tsp.
- Large spiralized zucchinis – 2
- Chopped cauliflower – 1 cup
- Garlic cloves – 2
- Small chopped onion – 1
- Large eggs – 2

Ingredients for the Seasoning:

- Ground smoked paprika - .5 tsp.
- Salt – 1 tsp.
- Black pepper - .5 tsp.
- Finely chopped chives – 1 tsp.
- Also Needed: Spiralizer

Preparation Method:

1. Rinse the zucchinis and discard the tips. Spiralize and set aside.
2. Plug in the Instant Pot. Give it a spritz of the olive oil in the stainless-steel insert. Add in the noodles and water and cook for 5 minutes. Set aside and cover.

3. Stir in the chopped cauliflower with a sprinkle of salt. Pour enough water to cover, and secure the top. Set the timer for 5 minutes using the high-pressure setting.
4. Quick release the pressure and add to the food processor with the salt, pepper, paprika, onion, and garlic. Blend until smooth.
5. Return the rest of the fixings into the Instant Pot and stir. Add the eggs on top and saute for around 3 minutes or until the eggs are cooked to your preference. Serve with a sprinkle of chives.

Chapter 3: lunch favorites

Whether you want some quick chicken, a bowl of soup or a salad; you'll find it here!

Chicken

Asian Turkey Stir-Fry

Freestyle Points: 2

Yields: 4 Servings

Ingredients:

- Asian vegetable mix - 16 oz. bag
- Ground turkey - 99% lean - 1 lb.
- Soy sauce – 4 tbsp.
- Minced cloves of garlic – 2
- Minced ginger – 2 tbsp.
- Coconut oil – 1 tbsp.
- Rice vinegar – 2 tbsp.
- Sesame oil – 1 tbsp.

Preparation Method:

1. Warm up the oil using med-high heat. Next, add the turkey, garlic, and ginger.
2. After the turkey is fully cooked; just dump the veggies into the pan. Next, cook it for 4 to 5 minutes or until tender.
3. Pour in the soy sauce and vinegar. Cook for two more minutes. Taste and add seasoning or soy sauce as desired before serving.

Buffalo Chicken Tenders

Freestyle Points: 5

Yields: 6 Servings

Ingredients:

- Chicken breasts – 1 lb.
- Panko breadcrumbs – 1 cup
- Flour - .25 cup
- Eggs – 3
- Red hot sauce - .33 cup
- Brown sugar - .5 cup
- Garlic powder - .5 tsp.
- Water – 3 tbsp.

Preparation Method:

1. Set the oven setting to 425°F.
2. Slice the chicken into strips and pound to 1/2-inch thickness for even cooking and tenderness. Toss into a zipper-type baggie along with the flour. Shake well.
3. Add the breadcrumbs in one dish and the eggs in another.
4. Dredge the chicken in the eggs, then the breadcrumbs. Arrange on a baking sheet and spray with a misting of cooking oil. Bake 20 minutes.
5. Prepare the sauce with the rest of the fixings in a small saucepan.
6. Enjoy the tenders with the sauce and your favorite side of veggies.

Salads

Caesar Salad – Instant Pot

Freestyle Points: 5

Yields: 5 Servings

Ingredients:

- Chicken breasts – 1 lb.
- Iceberg lettuce – 1 cup
- Pepper & Salt – to taste

Ingredients for the Dressing:

- Crushed garlic cloves - 2
- Greek yogurt - .25 cup
- Low-fat mayonnaise – 2 tsp.
- White wine vinegar – 1 tbsp.
- Freshly grated Italian Grana Padano cheese – 2 oz.

Preparation Method:

1. Combine the dressing fixings and set to the side.
2. Prepare the Instant Pot insert and spritz with some cooking oil. Warm it up using the saute function. Add the chicken with the pepper and salt. Saute three to four minutes per side. Take it out of the pot and set those aside also.
3. Roughly chop the lettuce and toss in the chicken with a sprinkle of the dressing.
4. Serve immediately and enjoy.

Ham Salad

Freestyle Points: 2

Yields: 4 Servings

Ingredients:

- Cooked – chopped ham – 1 cup
- Mango chutney – 1 tbsp.
- Onion powder – 2 tsp.
- Light mayonnaise – 2 tbsp.
- Dried mustard – 2 tsp.
- Non-fat plain Greek yogurt – 2 tbsp.

Preparation Method:

1. Pulse the fixings (omit the ham or not) in a processor until smooth.
2. Place the container in the refrigerator for about 30 minutes.
3. Add a dish of cucumber slices for a -0- points.

Pear & Blue Cheese Salad

Freestyle Points: 3

Servings: 4

Ingredients:

- White wine vinegar – 2 tbsp.
- Pear nectar - .25 cup
- Walnut oil – 2 tbsp.
- Ground black pepper - .125 tsp.
- Ground ginger - .125 tsp.
- Medium green pears – sliced - 3
- Torn mesclun greens – 10 cups
- Dijon mustard – 1 tsp.
- Honey – 1 tsp.
- Broken walnuts - .5 cup
- Crumbled blue cheese - .5 cup

Preparation Method:

1. Whisk the walnut oil, nectar, vinegar, honey, pepper, ginger, and mustard until well mixed. Set to the side for now.
2. Combine the rest of the ingredients and add the dressing. Toss well to coat. Chill in the fridge before time to eat.

Tuna Salad with Cranberries – Onion & Celery

Freestyle Points: 3

Yields: 5 Servings

Ingredients for the Seasoning – to taste:

- Red pepper flakes
- Freshly cracked black pepper
- Sea salt

Ingredients for the Tuna Salad:

- White tuna in spring water – 16 oz. can
- Low-fat mayonnaise – 3 tbsp.
- Light sour cream – 3 tbsp.
- Celery - .5 cup
- Red onion - .25 cup
- Dried cranberries - .25 cup
- Lemon juice – 1 tbsp.
- Cored apple - 1

Preparation Method:

1. Drain the tuna, mince the onion, and chop the celery. Core and thinly slice the apples.
2. Squeeze a fresh lemon for fresh juice. Combine the seasonings. Also, combine the salad fixings.
3. When ready to serve, garnish as desired and enjoy.

Soups

Beef Chili – Slow-Cooker

Freestyle Points: 4

Yields: 12 Servings

Ingredients:

- Lean ground beef – 1 lb.
- Diced bell peppers - 2
- Minced cloves of garlic
- Cumin – 2 tsp.
- Diced tomatoes – 1 can – 28 oz.
- Green chilis – canned .25 cup
- Kidney beans – 15 oz.
- Onion – 1 chopped
- Chili powder – 2 tbsp.
- Tomato paste – 2 tbsp.
- Salt – to taste

Preparation Method:

1. Warm up a skillet using the med-high temperature setting. Stir in the garlic and beef until browned (10 min. or so). Stir in the peppers and continue cooking 5 more minutes. Sprinkle with the cumin and chili powder.
2. Scoop the meat into the slow cooker with the remainder of the fixings. Stir and close the top. Prepare for eight to ten hours using the low-temperature setting.
3. When done, just taste test and adjust the seasonings to your liking.

Butternut Squash Soup

Freestyle Points: 1

Yields: 8 Servings

Ingredients:

- Raw cubed squash – 12 oz.
- Fat-free vegetable stock – 4 cups
- Green apple - .5 of 1
- Onion - .5 of 1
- Ground ginger – 1 pinch
- Black pepper & Salt – to taste
- Ground nutmeg – 1 pinch

Preparation Method:

1. Warm up a large stockpot and add the apple, onion, squash, and stock. Stir and cover until it boils. Then, reduce the temperature and remove the lid.
2. Continue cooking slowly for 10 minutes and puree with a blender. Give it a shake of salt, pepper, nutmeg, and ginger.
3. Serve and enjoy.

Chicken-Parmesan Soup

Freestyle Points: 3

Yields: 8 Servings

Ingredients:

- Olive oil – 1 tbsp.
- Minced cloves of garlic - 3
- Diced onion - 1
- Crushed tomatoes – 15 oz.
- Chicken stock – 6 cups
- Chicken breasts- no bones or skin – 12 oz.
- Part-skim mozzarella cheese – 1.5 cups
- Grated parmesan – 2 tbsp.
- Salt – 1 tsp.
- Red pepper flakes - .5 tsp.
- Dried parsley – 1 tsp.
- Black pepper - .5 tsp.

Preparation Method:

1. Prepare the stockpot using the med-high setting and add the oil. When warm, toss in the onions. Simmer 6 minutes. Toss in the garlic and continue cooking one additional minute.
2. Stir in the stock and tomatoes. Once it boils; just lower the heat setting. Remove the skin and bones from the chicken and add to the pot with the rest of the ingredients.
3. Simmer until the cheese is melted and serve.

Fish & Shrimp Stew

Freestyle Points: 2

Yields: 6 Servings

Ingredients:

- Minced garlic cloves - 2
- Crushed tomatoes – 28 oz. can
- Diced onion - 1
- Olive oil – 1 tbsp.
- Tomato paste – 3 tbsp.
- Parsley - .66 cup
- Fish stock – 14 oz.
- Clam juice – 8 oz.
- Ghee or butter – 2 tbsp.
- Basil – 5 tsp.
- Oregano - .5 tsp.
- Red pepper flakes - .25 tsp.
- Pepper and salt – to taste
- Raw shrimp – 1 lb.
- Cod – 2-inch pieces – 1.5 lb.

Preparation Method:

1. Use the medium heat setting to heat up the oil in a skillet. Toss in the onion and cook for five to seven minutes. Stir in the pepper flakes and garlic. Cook for another one to two minutes. Pour in the tomato paste and simmer one additional minute.
2. Stir in the tomatoes, clam juice, and fish stock. Simmer and add the basil, oregano, and butter. Simmer for 10-15 minutes.
3. Taste test and add the cod. Simmer for another 5 minutes and fold in the shrimp.
4. Continue cooking for 4-5 minutes until the shrimp is opaque.
5. Serve and enjoy.

Lentil Soup – Instant Pot

Freestyle Points: 1

Yield: 6 servings

Ingredients:

- Yellow onion - 1
- Carrots - 2
- Celery stalks - 2
- Diced tomatoes with juice – 1 can 15 oz.
- Garlic cloves - 2
- Curry powder – 1 tsp.
- Optional: Cayenne pepper - 1 pinch
- Ground cumin – 1 tsp.
- Dry green or brown lentils – 1 cup
- Water – 3 cups
- Freshly cracked black pepper – to taste
- Salt – 1 tsp. or more
- Fresh spinach - roughly chopped – 1 cup
- For Serving: Lemon slices

Preparation Method:

1. Plug in the Instant Pot to warm up for 10-15 minutes.
2. Peel and chop the onions, celery, and carrots. Mince the cloves of garlic and roughly chop the spinach.

3. Combine in the Instant Pot; the water, lentils, cayenne, curry, cumin, garlic, tomatoes, celery, onions, carrots, and a dash of black pepper. Stir well. (Omit the salt)
4. Close the top and lock it down. Set the timer for 10 minutes using the high-pressure setting. When it's done; just natural release the pressure for about 10 minutes and open the lid.
5. Stir and make sure the soup is well done. Add 1 teaspoon of salt with the spinach.
6. Serve warm after the spinach wilts. Garnish with a lemon wedge. Serve any time for up to a week when stored in the fridge in an airtight container.

Vegetable Soup

Freestyle Points: -0-

Yields: 6 Servings

Ingredients:

- Minced cloves of garlic - 3
- Chopped onion - 1
- Chicken stock - fat-free – 3 cups
- Frozen spinach – 10 oz.
- Diced zucchini - .5 cup
- Green beans - .5 cup
- Chopped carrots - .5 cup
- Tomato paste – 1 tbsp.
- Salt & Black pepper – to your liking
- Italian seasoning – 1 tsp.

Preparation Method:

1. Lightly spray a saucepan with some cooking oil spray. Warm it up using the medium heat setting and toss in the onion and garlic.
2. Cook about five minutes and stir in the tomato paste, stock, carrots, and green beans. Prepare for about 6 minutes.
3. Fold in the zucchini and simmer 5 additional minutes before adding the spinach to cook until heated.
4. Season to your liking and serve.

Chapter 4: scrumptious dinner choices: Beef – Fish & Seafood

Dinnertime is a special time of the day where your family can sit down and enjoy the conversations of daily events. From beef to fish and seafood, you will find a tempting dish to fit any occasion.

Beef Choices

Beef & Broccoli Stir-Fry

Freestyle Points: 3

Yields: 4 Servings

Ingredients:

- Lean sirloin beef - .75 lb.
- Table salt - .25 tsp.
- Cornstarch – divided – 2.5 tbsp.
- Canola oil – 2 tsp.
- Broccoli florets - 12 oz. bag – 5 cups
- Chicken broth – reduced-sodium – divided – 1 cup
- Minced garlic – 2 tbsp.
- Soy sauce - .25 cup
- Water - .25 cup
- Red pepper flakes - .25 tsp.
- Minced ginger root – 1 tbsp.

Preparation Method:

1. Combine two tablespoons of the cornstarch with the salt and add the beef to coat.
2. Warm up the oil in a wok or deep skillet using the med-hi heat setting.
3. Add the beef and cook for four minutes. Transfer to a bowl.
4. In the same pan, pour one-half cup of the broth and loosen the bits on the bottom. Fold in the broccoli and add one tbsp. of water - if needed. Cook for three minutes with the lid on.
5. Add the garlic, ginger, and pepper flakes. Simmer one more minute.
6. In a mixing cup, combine the rest of the broth, soy sauce, and remainder of the cornstarch. Pour into the pan and lower the temperature setting to med-low. Simmer one more minute and return the juices and beef into the pan. Toss to coat well and serve.

Beef & Mushrooms – Slow Cooker

Freestyle Points: 5

Yields: 6 Servings

Ingredients:

- Lean stewing beef meat – 2 lb.
- Olive oil – 2 tsp.
- Fresh mushrooms – 10 oz.
- Cream of mushroom soup – low-sodium/fat-free – 10.75 oz can
- Soup mix – dry onion – 1 envelope
- Dry red wine - .5 cup
- Suggested Cooker Size: 4-Quarts

Preparation Method:

1. Use the medium heat setting to warm up a skillet.
2. Do the Prep: Cube the stewing beef and slice the mushrooms.
3. Sprinkle the beef with the pepper and salt to your liking. Arrange it in the pan. Layer evenly and brown. Add to the cooker.
4. Brown the mushrooms and toss them into the pot.
5. Stir in the wine and scrape up the browned crunchies. Pour in the soup and soup mix. Mix well and cover.
6. Simmer on low for six to eight hours. Serve when ready.

Jalapeno Popper Burgers

Freestyle Points: 6

Yields: 4 Servings

Ingredients:

- 1 1/3 lb. ground beef – 1.33 lb.
- Finely chopped jalapeno - 1
- Cream cheese - reduced-fat – 2 tbsp.
- Mustard – 2 tsp.
- Worcestershire sauce – 2 tsp.
- Shredded cheddar cheese - .5 cup
- Kosher salt – divided – 5 tsp.

Preparation Method:

1. Combine all of the burger fixings. Divide into six patties and wait about 10 minutes before cooking for the flavors to mix.
2. Grill to your liking (4-6 min. per side suggested). If you prefer, use a skillet and cook for 5-6 minutes for each side.
3. Note: You can also use ground turkey.

Spicy Beef & Zucchini Skillet

Freestyle Points: 6

Yields: 4 Servings

Ingredients:

- Ground beef - lean – 1 lb.
- Olive oil – 1 tsp.
- Minced garlic cloves - 3
- Chopped onion - 1
- Green chilis - 1 can – 4 oz.
- Diced tomatoes - 14 oz. – 2 cans of each
- Drained black beans – 2 cans 14 oz. each
- Lime – juice of 1
- Chili powder – 1 tbsp.
- Chopped zucchinis - 2
- Ground black pepper & Salt – to taste

Preparation Method:

1. Use the med-high setting on the stovetop to heat up the oil.
2. Once it's hot, toss in the onions and garlic. Saute two minutes and add the beef. Once it is browning, stir in the chilis, beans, tomatoes, lime juice, chili powder, pepper, and salt.
3. Continue cooking for 10 minutes. Take off the top and add the chopped zucchini. Cook 10 more minutes and serve.

Fish & Seafood

Apple Trout

Freestyle Points: 3

Yields: 4 Servings

Ingredients:

- Soy sauce – 1 tsp.
- Freshly squeezed lemon juice – 1 tsp.
- Rice vinegar – 1 tsp.
- Granny Smith apple – 1 Medium
- Trout fillets – 7 oz.

Ingredients for the Seasoning Ingredients:

- Black pepper - .5 tsp
- Sea salt - .5 tsp
- Fresh parsley – 1 tbsp.
- Ground dried rosemary - .25 tsp.

Preparation Method:

1. Cut the apple and fillets into bite-sized pieces and squeeze the lemon juice.
2. Whisk the vinegar, lemon juice, soy sauce, rosemary, salt, pepper, and parsley in a mixing dish. Brush the trout.
3. Lightly grease the Instant Pot and add the oil. Using the saute function, add the apple and fish. Prepare 2 minutes. Add enough water to cover and secure the lid.
4. Set the timer for 2 minutes using the high-pressure setting. When the time is completed, open the lid and vent the steam.
5. Serve with your favorite 'zero' veggie.

Cajun Salmon

Freestyle Points: 1

Yields: 4 Servings

Ingredients:

- Olive oil – 1 tbsp.
- Salmon – 1.33 lb.
- Dried thyme - .25 tsp.
- Salt and Pepper - .5 tsp. each
- Paprika – 2 tsp.
- Onion powder - .5 tsp.
- Cayenne - .125 tsp.
- Garlic powder - .5 tsp.

Preparation Method:

1. Combine the spices to make the seasoning.
2. Brush the salmon with oil and a drizzle of the seasoning.
3. On the Grill: Arrange the salmon, so that the skin is facing downwards. Cook three to four minutes. Turn the salmon over and continue cooking for an additional 1-3 minutes. Choose a delicious side dish and serve.

Chapter 5: scrumptious dinner choices: Pork & poultry

Pork

Cuban Pork – Instant Pot

Freestyle Points: 5

Yields: 10 Servings

Ingredients:

- Garlic cloves – 6
- Pork shoulder blade roast – boneless – 3 lb.
- Bay leaf – 1
- Kosher salt – 1 tbsp.
- Lime juice - .66 cup
- Grapefruit juice- .66 cup
- Fresh oregano – 5 tbsp.
- Cumin – 5 tbsp.

Ingredients for Serving:

- Salsa
- Lime wedges
- Chopped cilantro
- Hot sauce
- Tortillas

Preparation Method:

1. Chop the meat into four pieces and place in a mixing container.
2. Use a mini food processor and combine both of the juices, garlic, salt, cumin, and oregano. Blend until smooth.
3. Pour the mixture over the shoulder pieces and let it marinate one hour on the countertop. You can also marinate overnight in the refrigerator.
4. When ready to prepare; add the meat to the cooker along with the bay leaf.
5. Cook using the high-pressure setting for 80 minutes. Natural release the pressure.
6. Shred the meat and remove the juices from the Instant Pot/pressure cooker.
7. Pour one cup of the juices and add the meat back into the pot. Season to taste. Keep it warm until serving time.

Pork Chops with Creamy Sauce

Freestyle Points: 5

Yields: 4 Servings

Ingredients:

- Pork loin chops - center-cut – 4 - Approximately 4 oz. ea.
- Non-fat Half-and-Half - .33 cup
- Fat-free chicken stock - .33 cup
- Black pepper - .5 tsp.
- Onion powder - .5 tsp.
- Salt - .5 tsp.
- Dijon mustard – 1.5 tbsp.
- Dried thyme – 1 pinch

Preparation Method:

1. Shake the salt, pepper, and onion powder over the chops.
2. Using the med-high heat setting on the stovetop, prepare a large skillet with cooking spray.
3. Once the pan is hot, add the chops and fry for 3-4 minutes per side. The internal temperature should reach a minimum temperature on a meat thermometer of 145°F.
4. At this point; just place the prepared chops in a closed container and keep them warm.
5. Pour the chicken stock into the skillet and deglaze the browned bits. Stir in the mustard and Half-and-Half.
6. Lower the temperature setting to medium and continue cooking for 7 minutes. When the sauce has thickened, add the thyme.
7. Serve with the sauce and your favorite side dish.

Raspberry Pork Chops in the Crock Pot

Freestyle Points: 8

Yields: 4 servings

Ingredients:

- Boneless pork chops – 4 – 4 oz. each
- Seasonings: Pepper – salt – meat seasoning; ex. Montreal Steak
- Chicken broth - .25 cup
- Raspberry jam - .75 cup
- Balsamic vinegar – 3 tbsp.
- Chopped chipotle pepper in adobo sauce – 1 tsp.
- Suggested Cooker Size: 4-quarts

Preparation Method:

1. Lightly grease the slow cooker. Whisk the finely chopped chipotle, vinegar, broth, and jam.
2. Season the pork chops to your liking and add two of them to the cooker. Add the sauce and the last two chops with the rest of the sauce.
3. Secure the top and cook 4-6 hours on the low setting.
4. Enjoy with a salad or dish of brown rice.

Poultry

Cheesy Southwestern Chicken – Slow Cooker

Freestyle Points: 1

Yields: 6 Servings

Ingredients:

- Chunky salsa – 16 oz. – 1 jar - divided
- Chicken breast halves - 6
- Corn – 15.5 oz. ea. – 2 cans
- Black beans - 15 oz. – 1 can
- Low-fat shredded Mexican cheese blend – 1 cup
- Optional: Southwest seasoning blend
- Suggested: 5-6-quart slow cooker

Preparation Method:

1. Rinse and drain the corn and black beans. Add to the slow cooker with about half of the salsa.
2. Remove the bones and skin from the chicken. Shake with the salt and pepper or seasoning blend if using.
3. Add the chicken to the pot and the rest of the salsa. Secure the lid and cook on the low-temperature setting until tender (4-6 hrs.).
4. Sprinkle with the cheese. Cover again to melt the cheese (5 min.).

Italian – Balsamic Chicken

Freestyle Points: 1

Yields: 4 Servings

Ingredients:

- Breasts of chicken – 1.33 lb.
- Salt and pepper – 1 tsp. each
- Italian seasoning – 2 tsp.
- Balsamic vinegar – 2.5 tbsp.
- Olive oil – 2 tsp.
- Minced garlic cloves - 3
- Sliced mushrooms - 8 oz.
- Chicken stock - .5 cup

Preparation Method:

1. Combine the salt, pepper, and Italian seasoning. Sprinkle the chicken.
2. Warm up a skillet with the oil using the med-high heat setting. When ready, add the seasoned chicken. Simmer slowly for two to three minutes on each side. Put it to the side for now.
3. Toss the garlic and mushrooms into the pan and saute three to four minutes. Stir in the vinegar and chicken stock. Stir well and deglaze the pan. Toss the chicken in the sauce and simmer about 10 to 15 minutes until done.
4. Note: Be sure to use high-quality balsamic vinegar for the best results.

Oven-Baked Chicken Kebabs – Slow Cooker

Freestyle Points: 2

Yields: 4 Servings

Ingredients:

- Olive oil – 2 tbsp.
- Fresh parsley - .25 cup
- Taco seasoning – 1 tsp.
- Salt – 1 tsp.
- Minced cloves of garlic - 3
- Boneless chicken breasts – 1.33 lb.
- Yellow - red or mixed bell peppers - 2
- Cherry tomatoes – a small handful
- Onion – 1 small
- Juiced limes - 2

Preparation Method:

1. Cut the onion and peppers into chunks. Juice the lime.
2. Add the taco seasoning, salt, garlic, oil, juice of the lime, and parsley in a blender. Process until it's smooth.
3. Cube the chicken and shake in the bag of prepared marinade. Store in the fridge for about 30 minutes.
4. When ready to prepare, warm up the oven broiler.
5. Arrange the chicken tomatoes, peppers, and onions on skewers.
6. Add the prepared kebabs onto a baking tin.
7. Bake for 5 minutes and flip. Broil for another 5 minutes.
8. Serve when the chicken reaches an internal temperature of 165°F.
9. Note: You can add other fixings to the kebabs if you have some extras on hand. (Be sure to check for any additional points.)

Pesto Baked Chicken

Freestyle Points: 3

Yields: 4 Servings

What You Need:

- Butterflied chicken breasts – 1 lb.
- Pesto - .25 cup
- Low-fat grated mozzarella cheese - .5 cup
- Cherry tomatoes- 1 cup
- Sea salt & Freshly cracked black pepper – to your liking

Preparation Method:

1. Cut away all of the bones and skin from the chicken. Slice the tomatoes into halves.
2. Warm up the oven to 400°F. Prepare a baking tin with a sheet of aluminum foil and a spritz of non-stick spray.
3. Coat with the pepper and salt with a spread of the pesto.
4. Place on the baking tin with the tomatoes. Bake 15-17 minutes.
5. Take it out of the oven and drizzle with the cheese. Bake another 5-6 minutes until the cheese is lightly browned.

Chapter 6: Delicious sides

Pair off one of these delicious dishes with your main course.

Sides

Asparagus Sauteed with Bacon

Freestyle Points: 1

Yields: 4 Servings – .66 cup each

Ingredients:

- Medium sliced shallot - 1
- Asparagus – 1 lb.
- Sea salt - .25 tsp.
- Freshly cracked black pepper - .125 tsp.
- Center-cut bacon – 4 slices
- White wine vinegar – 1.5 tsp.

Preparation Method:

6. Slice the bacon into small pieces. Prepare in a skillet for 5 minutes. Remove and drain on a paper towel. Leave only one teaspoon of grease in the pan and pour the rest in a jar for later or discard.
7. Trim and dice the asparagus into chunks and slice the shallots. Add to the pan and saute about 7 minutes, stirring frequently.
8. Toss the bacon, pepper, and salt over the mixture using the med-high temperature until warm.
1. Transfer to serving dishes and stir in the vinegar.

Brown Sugar Baked Beans – Instant Pot

Freestyle Points: 2

Yield: 8 servings

Ingredients:

- Finely diced yellow onion - 1
- Northern beans -approx. 1.75 cups
- Kidney beans - 1 can – 15.5 oz. - approx. 1.75 cups
- Pinto beans - 1 can or approx. 1.75 cups
- Chili powder - 1 tsp.
- Water - .75 cup
- Ketchup - .5 cup
- Dark brown sugar – not packed - .33 cup
- Yellow mustard – 1 tbsp.

Preparation Method:

9. Rinse and drain the beans. Combine all of the fixings in the Instant Pot. Secure the lid and lock. Use the manual setting on high-pressure for 8 minutes.
1. Natural release the pressure when the time has elapsed (10-15 minutes) or quick release if you are in a hurry. Stir before serving.

Caesar Green Beans

Freestyle Points: 2

Yields: 4 Servings

Ingredients for the Beans:

- Water – 2 cups
- Green beans – 1 lb.
- Low-cal Caesar dressing – 1.5 tbsp.
- Shredded parmesan cheese – 1 tbsp.

Ingredients for the Crumb Topping:

- Powdered garlic – 1 tsp.
- Low-cal butter – 1 tsp.
- Whole grain toast – 1 slice

Preparation Method:

1. Trim the green beans and shred the cheese.
2. Toss the greens into a pot of boiling water. Simmer until tender (5 min.). Add to a colander to remove the liquids.
3. Butter the toast and sprinkle with the garlic. Microwave 10 minutes and add to a food processor. Blitz until crumbly.
4. Serve the beans with a sprinkle of the crumbs and a serving of dressing. Sprinkle with the parmesan and serve.

Creamy Broccoli – Instant Pot

Freestyle Points – 4

Yields: 4 Servings

Ingredients:

- Vegetable stock – 2 cups
- Chopped broccoli – 1 lb.
- Halved brussels sprouts – 1 cup
- Sliced red onion – 1 medium-sized
- Minced cloves of garlic – 2
- Salt - .5 tsp.

Ingredients for the Sauce:

- Soy sauce – 1 tbsp.
- Freshly squeezed lime juice – 1 tsp.
- Heavy cream – 2 tbsp.
- Olive oil – 1 tbsp.
- Ground black pepper & salt - .5 tsp. each
- Freshly ground ginger - .25 tsp.
- Also Needed: Food Processor

Preparation Method:

5. Add the brussels sprouts and broccoli to the stainless-steel insert of the Instant Pot. Pour in the vegetable stock and salt.
6. Close the lid and choose the high-pressure setting for five minutes.
7. When the timer buzzes, quick release the pressure and remove the veggies with a slotted spoon.
8. Prep the food processor by adding the garlic, onions, and each of the sauce fixings. Pulse until the mixture is creamy.
9. Select the saute function and pour the prepared sauce into the insert. Let it simmer for five minutes. Stir occasionally.
1. Serve over the veggies and enjoy!

Mashed Sweet Potatoes

Freestyle Points: 2

Servings: 4

Ingredients:

- Large sweet potatoes - 2
- Salt & Black pepper - .5 tsp of each
- Garlic powder – 1 tsp.
- Plain fat-free Greek yogurt - .5 cup

Preparation Method:

1. Wash, peel, and cube the potatoes. Prepare a pot of boiling water (enough to cover the potatoes). Add the potatoes. Boil using the med-high stovetop setting for 8-10 minutes.
2. Dump the potatoes into a colander to drain and add to a large mixing container. Combine with the seasonings and yogurt.
3. Use a hand mixer or mix by hand to mash the fixings until smooth.

Pinto Beans - Crockpot

Freestyle Points: -0-

Yields: 8 Servings

Ingredients:

- Onion - 1
- Dry pinto beans – 1 lb.
- Bay leaves - 2
- Garlic cloves - 4
- Poblano peppers - 2
- Salt – 1 tsp.
- Cumin - .5 tbsp.
- Water or broth – to cover the beans – 6 cups

Preparation Method:

1. Dice the garlic, peppers, and onion. Rinse the beans thoroughly and add to the crockpot.
2. Toss in the rest of the fixings and cover with broth or water. It should be at least one inch over the beans.
3. Prepare for 8-10 hours using the low setting. Times vary with each cooker. When done, the beans will be soft and tasty.

Rainbow Potato Salad

Freestyle Points: 4

Yields: 6 Servings

Ingredients for the Potatoes:

- Yellow potatoes – 1 lb.
- Purple potatoes - .5 lb.
- Red potatoes - .5 lb.

Ingredients for the Dressing:

- Fresh dill - .5 cup
- Scallions - .5 cup
- Celery – 1 stalk
- Low-calorie ranch dressing - .5 cup
- Salt and pepper – to taste

Preparation Method:

1. Cube the potatoes. Finely chop the scallions and celery. Roughly chop the dill.
2. Add all of the potatoes to a pan full of water. Boil and cover. Continue to cook until softened (10-12 min.).
3. Drain the water out of the potatoes and let cool.
4. Combine the dressing fixings in a mixing container. When cool, add the potatoes and stir until incorporated.
5. Chill in the fridge or serve warm.

Roasted Carrots

Freestyle Points: 2

Yields: 4 Servings

Ingredients:

- Baby carrots - 1 bag – 16 oz.
- Dried parsley - .25 tsp.
- Salt - .25 tsp.
- Black pepper – 1 pinch
- Ginger - .25 tsp.
- Cinnamon – 1 pinch
- Olive oil – 1.5 tbsp.
- Also Needed: 9 x 13 casserole dish

Preparation Method:

1. Warm up the oven to 450°F.
2. Prepare the baking dish with the oil and carrots. Sprinkle with the fixings. Bake for 20-25 minutes until tender.
3. Serve with your favorite main dish.

In the next segment, you will discover how easy it is to prepare a days-worth of meals and stay within your desired goals. Once you know how many points you can add to your menu plan (your personal total of allowed points), feel free to add up to those limits and enjoy the freedom provided by your new way of life. Each day has the total provided for points allowed for each recipe item and a daily total.

Chapter 7: 21-day meal plan

DAY 1:

- Breakfast: Baked Omelet – 2
- Lunch: Fish & Shrimp Stew – 2
- Dinner: Beef & Broccoli Stir-Fry – 3

Totals - Day 1: 7

DAY 2:

- Breakfast: Banana Roll-Ups – 2
- Lunch: Buffalo Chicken Tenders – 5
- Lunch Side: Asparagus Sauteed with Bacon – 1
- Dinner: Apple Trout – 3
- Dinner: Side: Brown Sugar Baked Beans – Instant Pot - 2

Totals – Day 2: 13

DAY 3:

- Breakfast: Broccoli Cheddar Egg Muffins - 2
- Lunch: Caesar Salad – Instant Pot – 5
- Dinner: Cheesy Southwestern Chicken – Slow Cooker -1
- Dinner Side: Rainbow Potato Salad – 4

Totals - Day 3: 12

DAY 4:

- Breakfast: Cinnamon-Apple French Toast – 4
- Lunch: Asian Turkey Stir-Fry - 2
- Dinner: Cuban Pork – Instant Pot – 5

- Dinner Side: Pinto Beans – Crockpot - 0-

Totals - Day 4: 11

DAY 5:

- Breakfast: Country Cottage Pancakes – 3
- Lunch: Ham Salad – 2
- Lunch Side: Caesar Green Beans – 2
- Dinner: Beef & Mushrooms – Slow Cooker – 5
- Dinner Side: Roasted Carrots - 2

Totals - Day 5: 14

DAY 6:

- Breakfast: Egg & Sausage Muffins – 1
- Lunch: Pear & Blue Cheese Salad - 3
- Dinner: Cajun Salmon – 1
- Dinner Side: Fully-Loaded Macaroni & Cheese with Veggies – 6

Totals - Day 6: 11

DAY 7:

- Breakfast: Egg & Veggie Scramble - 1
- Lunch: Butternut Squash Soup – 1
- Dinner: Jalapeno Popper Burgers – 6

Totals - Day 7: 8

DAY 8:

- Breakfast: Hard-Boiled Eggs in the Instant Pot -0-

- Lunch: Beef Chili – Slow-Cooker - 4
- Dinner: Italian – Balsamic Chicken – 1
- Dinner Side: Leftover - Dinner Side: Fully-Loaded Macaroni & Cheese with Veggies – 6

Totals - Day 8: 11

DAY 9:

- Breakfast: Tropical Breakfast Pie – 5
- Lunch: Asian Turkey Stir-Fry - 2
- Dinner: Italian – Balsamic Chicken – 1
- Dinner Side: Mashed Sweet Potatoes - 2

Totals - Day 9: 10

DAY 10:

- Breakfast: Muffin Tin Eggs – 1
- Lunch: Chicken-Parmesan Soup – 3
- Dinner: Spicy Beef & Zucchini Skillet - 6

Totals - Day 10: 10

DAY 11:

- Breakfast: Zucchini Noodles & Poached Eggs - 4
- Lunch: Tuna Salad with Cranberries – Onion & Celery - 3
- Dinner: Pork Chops with Creamy Sauce – 5
- Dinner Side: Roasted Carrots - 2

Totals – Day 11: 14

DAY 12:

- Breakfast: Baked Omelet – 2
- Lunch: Lentil Soup – Instant Pot – 1
- Dinner: Oven-Baked Chicken Kebabs – Slow Cooker – 2
- Dinner Side: Asparagus Sauteed with Bacon - 1

Totals - Day 12: 6

DAY 13:

- Breakfast: Egg & Sausage Muffins – 1
- Lunch: Fish & Shrimp Stew - 2
- Dinner: Pork Chops with Creamy Sauce – 5
- Dinner Side: Mashed Sweet Potatoes - 2

Totals - Day 13: 10

DAY 14:

- Breakfast: Broccoli Cheddar Egg Muffins - 2
- Lunch: Ham Salad - 2
- Dinner: Pesto Baked Chicken – 3
- Dinner Side: Creamy Broccoli – Instant Pot - 4

Totals - Day 14: 11

DAY 15:

- Breakfast: Banana Roll-Ups – 2
- Lunch: Vegetable Soup -0-
- Dinner: Raspberry Pork Chops in the Crock Pot – 8
- Dinner Side: Caesar Green Beans - 2

Totals - Day 15: 12

DAY 16:

- Breakfast: Cinnamon-Apple French Toast – 4
- Lunch: Butternut Squash Soup – 1
- Dinner: Apple Trout – 3
- Dinner Side: Brown Sugar Baked Beans – Instant Pot - 2

Totals - Day 16: 10

DAY 17:

- Breakfast: Muffin Tin Eggs – 1
- Lunch: Tuna Salad with Cranberries – Onion & Celery - 3
- Dinner: Beef & Broccoli Stir-Fry – 3

Totals - Day 17: 7

DAY 18:

- Breakfast: Egg & Veggie Scramble - 1
- Lunch: Buffalo Chicken Tenders - 5
- Dinner: Cuban Pork – Instant Pot – 5

Totals - Day 18: 11

DAY 19:

- Breakfast: Breakfast: Hard-Boiled Eggs in the Instant Pot –0–
- Lunch: Pear & Blue Cheese Salad - 3
- Dinner: Spicy Beef & Zucchini Skillet - 6

Totals - Day 19: 9

DAY 20:

- Breakfast: Tropical Breakfast Pie – 5
- Lunch: Beef Chili – Slow-Cooker - 4
- Dinner: Oven-Baked Chicken Kebabs – Slow Cooker – 2
- Dinner Side: Creamy Broccoli – Instant Pot - 4

Totals - Day 20: 15

DAY 21:

- Breakfast: Country Cottage Pancakes - 3
- Lunch: Caesar Salad – Instant Pot – 5
- Dinner: Cajun Salmon – 1
- Dinner Side: Rainbow Side Salad - 4

Totals - Day 21: 13

Now, just continue with the same pattern and add up to your daily number of Freestyle points. These are just your basic meals; so, enjoy the rest of the points but use them wisely each day.

www.ingramcontent.com/pod-product-compliance
Lightning Source LLC
Chambersburg PA
CBHW071610080526
44588CB00010B/1079